Current Health Policy Issues and Alternatives

Current Health Policy Issues and Alternatives

An Applied Social Science Perspective

Carole E. Hill, Editor

Southern Anthropological Society Proceedings, No. 19
Mary W. Helms, Series Editor

The University of Georgia Press
Athens and London

Southern Anthropological Society

Founded 1966

© 1986 by the Southern Anthropological Society
Published by the University of Georgia Press
Athens, Georgia 30602
All rights reserved

Set in 11 on 13 Times Roman
The paper in this book meets the guidelines for permanence and durability of the Committee on Production Guidelines for Book Longevity of the Council on Library Resources.

Printed in the United States of America

90 89 88 87 86   5 4 3 2 1

Library of Congress Cataloging in Publication Data

Current health policy issues and alternatives.

(Southern Anthropological Society proceedings;
no. 19)
"Most of the papers in this volume were delivered
in the key symposium of the 1984 annual meeting of
the Southern Anthropological Society, held in
Atlanta, Georgia"—Introd.
Bibliography: p.
1. Medical policy—Social aspects—United States—
Congresses. 2. Medical policy—Social aspects—
Congresses. I. Hill, Carole E. II. Southern
Anthropological Society. Meeting (19th: 1984:
Atlanta, Ga.) III. Series. [DNLM: 1. Delivery of
Health Care—congresses. 2. Health Planning—
congresses. 3. Health Policy—congresses.
W1 S093K no. 19 / WA 540.1 C976 1984]
GN2.S9243 no. 19 [RA395] 301s [362.1′042] 86-4303
ISBN 0-8203-0868-4 (alk. paper)
ISBN 0-8203-0869-2 (pbk.: alk. paper)

Contents

Current Health Policy Issues and Alternatives

Introduction

Carole E. Hill

Social scientists are increasingly becoming involved in the development, implementation, and evaluation of health policy and programs. Health policies guide the parameters of organized health services and programs of change and, at the same time, reflect the structure and culture of a society. The implementation of policies and programs are carried out in communities and neighborhoods whose culture and structure may vary with that of the policymakers. Consequently, social scientists working in health policy must examine the macrolevel of policymaking and the microlevel of policy implementation in the local level.

This volume is concerned with the intersection of current health policy issues with the approaches of applied social science for the purpose of delineating alternative policies for health care organization and delivery. Each paper utilizes original research as data bases for suggesting changes in current health policies. Each addresses a policy issue and using empirical data suggests alternative ways to intervene in and solve health care problems in a variety of settings. Although four papers focus on populations outside the United States, all deal with current national and international health policies of the U.S. government. Therefore, for the sake of continuity, each author was asked to use the writings of Robert Alford as a guideline for his or her policy discussion. According to Alford (1972), there are at least three perspectives that have affected health policy in the United States—market reformers (expansionists and laissez-faire), equal rights reformers, and bureaucratic reformers. They all include distinct values concerning economic, social, and political reform and as a consequence have different impacts on the organization and delivery of health service to a population. A report of the Rockefeller Foundation concurs with Alford by stating that "health care policies reflect the cultural, social, economic and political characteristics of a state" (Evans 1981:12).

Furthermore, in his book *Health Care Politics,* Alford discusses the consequences of health research and states that "little systematic knowledge exists about the ways in which the present health care system works or the alternatives that might be feasible. Not only are basic descriptive data scarce, but relevant research on the system as a whole has not been done" (1975:239). His primary concern is the "ways in which ideologies are constructed to defend structural intersets composed of clusters of social roles and positions attached to only parts of individuals" (1975:18–19) while assuming "that there is a reasonably high correlation between ideologies and personal incentives of doctors, researchers, administrators and the organizational interests of medical professors, hospitals or public health associations" (1975:21). Most of the papers address these issues and several suggest that programs have failed because of lack of congruity with the culture and structure of impacted populations. They suggest creative alternatives to current policies that will take the ideologies of culturally different populations into consideration. Indeed, this is the crux of an applied social science perspective: an objective and relativistic perspective in solving human health problems cross-culturally.

The policy problems addressed in this volume deal with environmental health, mental health, primary health care, ethnicity and health care, health education, dietary strategies, and traditional medicine. Although most of the papers are written by anthropologists, they all take an interdisciplinary perspective and discuss policy issues within a broader context than that of just one discipline. The paper by Thompson provides a framework for subsequent discussions. He suggests that social scientists, particularly anthropologists, must consider the health policy context if they are to be more relevant to the deliberations of policymakers. By sketching some dominant characteristics of health policy in contemporary Western democracies, he demonstrates the close relationship between these issues and the health policy and political questions in the development of Third World countries (the politics of breakthrough). In general, he feels that policymakers have difficulty understanding the complexity of cultural issues.

These observations are especially illustrated in the papers by Gordon and Robillard. Gordon examines the problems extant in the delivery of mental health services to Hispanic groups in a New England city. While emphasizing alcoholism, he suggests that one of the major problems in successful treatment involves the cultural versus the medical perspective. Bureaucratic reform is not the answer to solving the alcoholic problems of these groups; the cultural constraints to the medical model appear to be the major reason for the failure of the program. Likewise, Robillard discusses the cultural problems that arose when programs based on a Western ideology of mental health attempted to "upgrade" the mental health of the indigenous peoples of Micronesia. His evaluation of the eleven programs reveals that assumptions of individualism, capitalism and underlying purposes of the world economic and political development policies contribute to their failure. He suggests a model of interorganizational linkages that will bring social scientists together with policymakers to hopefully avoid such ignorance in future programs for the purpose of designing more culturally appropriate health services.

The nutritional status of a population is inextricably linked to that country's agricultural policies. In her paper, DeWalt examines the dietary correlates of changing agricultural strategies in a Mexican community and argues that the change from subsistence agriculture to cash cropping has resulted in a change in the dietary behavior of farmers. Through linking these national policies to the household level in a community, DeWalt demonstrates that policy changes that emphasize cash crops over subsistence crops do not necessarily make for a "better diet" and, indeed, can result in a loss of food security on the household level. In order to increase nutritional status, she suggests several alternative nutritional strategies within the context of agricultural policies in Mexico. Again, we are able to clearly see the importance of assessing the health impacts of national policies on the local level.

New and Cheung discuss a trend in China contrary to these recommendations. Although the Communist Revolution supported the training of traditional healers and fostered a respect for the traditional health system, in recent years the scientific medical system has become the dominant model for training and service delivery. The authors take us through a history of the relationship of these two systems of medicine and conclude that integration is still only a dream of anthropologists and other social scientists who take a more holistic perspective.

In her paper that compares the primary health care system in Costa Rica with that of the United States, Hill suggests policy alternatives that would involve the community in the planning and implementation process. Both systems, although different in design, are still based primarily on a curative rather than a preventive model of health care, a major obstacle for developing a primary health care program. Emphasis on community involvement is also the focus of Couto's paper. He goes further, however, by framing his discussions and critique of environmental health and epidemiology within the context of science versus politics and personal knowledge versus scientific knowledge. His suggestions for changing environmental health research policy are revolutionary and, like Hill, Couto calls for major alterations in the current structure and culture of health planning, policy, and research.

Heeding the advice of Thompson—that social scientists should look at the policy context—Angrosino and Whiteford ask a seemingly obvious albeit very complicated question: "How is health policy made?" They suggest that decision making is a very small part of the policy process and proceed to illustrate, through examining policy initiatives in two case studies, the role of an agency in an advocacy policy process. Similar to the paper by Couto, they argue that innovation and creativity can stem from the local structures and informal linkages with an agency which can initiate policy rather than just implement it.

The last two papers discuss the impact of social science in international health policy and contemplate policy conflicts and change for future public health education. Both paint a rather dim picture of the extent that social scientists, and particularly the anthropological perspective, have been used in health policy and health education. Bloom presents the "inside perspective" by discussing her experience in the Health Policy Section of the Agency for International Development. After setting forth the general policy process, she suggests ways in which anthropologists can play larger roles in this process. She is an optimist for the future of anthropology in health policy. While not as optimistic, Strauss and Conrad, public health educators, discuss the organization and the contemporary political issues in education and public health and suggest that the social science content of the public health curricula should be expanded. They feel that if public health is to obtain its stated goals, a more holistic perspective must be taken in health education policy.

So, we end as we began, but with an inverted look at health policy and social science. Thompson tells us not to forget the policy context, while we know that this context is a reflection of the social and cultural structures and ideology in which they are found. As several of the papers illustrate, however, they reflect the dominant structure and culture while often ignoring alternative perspectives on the nature of health and health services. Two of the papers nonetheless demonstrate that the people who represent these alternative viewpoints can affect policy. All the papers illustrate that policymakers should not ignore the social and cultural context of health, health policy, and health education.

Most of the papers in this volume were delivered in the Key Symposium of the 1984 annual meeting of the Southern Anthropological Society held in Atlanta, Georgia. There are several people to whom I would like to express my appreciation in helping me organize the symposium and subsequently helping to finalize the manuscript. Ivia Cofresi kept me organized and tracked down references; Susan Hamilton, with her usual efficiency, organized the references; and Stephen Fievet diligently retyped several of the papers. Finally, I would like to thank the participants in the Key Symposium for cooperating with the deadlines and working with me on the editorial changes.

The Health Policy Context

Frank J. Thompson

What can anthropologists contribute to efforts to delineate alternative policies for health care organization and delivery? As a political scientist looking at the question from outside the discipline, I feel they can contribute a great deal. More than other social scientists, anthropologists have remained sensitive to the importance of enthnographic methods of research. These methods can legitimately claim a significant place in the research repertoire needed to analyze the development, evolution, and outcomes of public programs (Van Maanen 1983; Williams 1982). Furthermore, anthropologists have usually focused on the grass roots of the policy system—the community in which some health service or benefit gets delivered. This propensity serves as a useful corrective for the centralist and often simplistic perspectives of those who dominate policymaking networks in the capitols of countries.

As anthropologists strive to become more relevant to the deliberations of policymakers, it is important that they consider the health policy context. This essay provides a backdrop for the more specific papers that follow. In particular, it sketches some dominant characteristics of health policies in contemporary Western democracies, especially the United States. It then briefly juxtaposes fundamental policy and political questions raised by developments in the Third World. Finally, and in light of this description, it returns to the importance of applied anthropology for those who would develop more sensible health policies.

TECHNICAL POLITICS IN THE INDUSTRIALIZED DEMOCRACIES

The 1960s and 1970s witnessed major developments in health policy in the industrialized democracies, particularly the United States. These developments pertain to two major types of policies, preventive and medical. Preventive policies aim beyond the confines of the medical service model. They proceed under the banner of fighting death and disease by striving to reduce health hazards in the environment or by modifying personal life-styles detrimental to health. In this regard, the proliferation of a host of regulatory policies aimed at exorcising health hazards from the environment has been a particularly conspicuous development. In the United States, for instance, Congress passed such laws as the Clean Air Act Amendments of 1970, the Occupational Safety and Health Act of 1970, and the Safe Drinking Water Act of 1974. Important and controversial as many of these preventive policies are, they garner a much smaller portion of the public sector's investment in health than medical policies.

Medical policies seek to alter access to health care, its cost, or its quality. During the last twenty years the United States became more like Europe in assuring access to medical care, although the percentage of health expenditures paid for by the public sector amounted to just over 40 percent, roughly half of that common in most European countries (U.S. Public Health Service 1983:266). Pivotal developments in the United States occurred in 1965 when Congress approved medical programs for the elderly (Medicare) and the poor (Medicaid). These programs along with other initiatives appeared to improve access to health care for many groups, particularly the poor. From 1964 to 1981, for instance, physician visits per person per year increased from 3.9 to 5.6 among members of the lowest income bracket. During the same period, the total number of physician visits per person remained constant at 4.6 (U.S. Public Health Service 1983:219). Statistics such as these hardly meant that governments had solved all problems of access. Since the poor have more health problems than other income groups, questions lingered as to whether the poor received as much treatment as they needed. A small segment of the population remained without any health insurance coverage whatsoever. On balance, however, the United States became more like other industrialized democracies in striking down many barriers to health care.

Whatever problems of access to medical care persisted, these problems increasingly took a back seat to issues of cost in the United States and Western Europe during the 1970s. Policymakers seized upon several indicators to argue that health care expenditures had mushroomed out of control. The United States, for instance, witnessed a steady increase in national health expenditures as a percentage of the gross national product—from 5.3 percent in 1960 to 10.5 percent in 1982. The price of medical care more than tripled in the period from 1965 through 1981. Energy prices comprised the only component of the consumer price index to rise at a more rapid rate. Health care outlays also began to put major strains on government budgets. Medicare costs, for instance, rose from $4.5 billion in fiscal 1967 to an estimated $70 billion in 1985 (U.S. Office of Management and Budget 1984; U.S. Public Health Service 1983:259, 263, 280).

As issues of cost loomed increasingly large, the United States joined other Western democracies in moving from breakthrough politics toward technical politics.[1] The former kind of politics revolves around basic reforms where government considers or launches new initiatives that presage substantial change in its role in the medical sector. The struggle leading to the passage of Medicare legislation serves as an example (Marmor 1970). Technical politics, by contrast, involves efforts to repair or rationalize programs already in operation. The ongoing debate over how to redesign payment systems for medical providers that will increase their incentive to deliver cost-effective care provides an obvious illustration.

Politics becomes more technical to the degree that it features three basic properties. First, its technical character increases to the extent that debates tend to be couched in terms of economy, efficiency, adjustment, and repair rather than ideological rhetoric that distinguishes the Left from the Right on the political spectrum. Unlike the politics of breakthrough, technical politics does not feature clashes over basic boundary issues of whether government ought to be involved in some policy arena. Even political leaders with long-standing credentials as conservative ideologues, such as Mrs. Thatcher and Mr. Reagan, do not publicly quarrel with the idea that government should take steps to ensure access to health care for key groups in society. Instead, they seek to chip away at these programs through marginal adjustment and retreat. Those at the other end of the political spectrum tend to abandon energetic pursuit of fundamental reform in health care. Comprehensive national health insurance has, for instance, ceased to be a major priority for the Democratic party in the United States. Instead, these political leaders tend to spend their time scrutinizing proposed policy adjustments to determine whether they would recreate past inequities in access to medical care. Their quest for greater cost-effectiveness frequently focuses on limiting the excesses of medical providers.

Despite its emphasis on marginal adjustment, technical politics is by no means trivial politics. Relatively small changes in the procedures for paying hospitals can, for instance, undercut their incentive to serve the poor. Furthermore, many small changes can over time have a large impact. While technical politics can profoundly shape who gets what from government in the health arena, the language of this politics emphasizes tinkering and the rationalization of existing programs.

Second, politics becomes technical to the degree that the issues it addresses pose complexities that the media and the populace cannot readily grasp. The politics of breakthrough tends to feature large questions that the media can dramatize and ordinary citizens believe they can understand. Should the federal government assure access to medical care for all citizens? For the elderly? For the poor? Many citizens believe that they can comprehend the issues these questions raise and feel confident about answering them. In contrast, the questions of technical politics are usually far more abstruse. Should the new hospital payment system for Medicare based on Diagnosis Related Groups (DRGs) be extended to all third-party payors, i.e., to hospital reimbursements by both government and private insurance companies? If one can imagine doing a street poll on this subject, it is easy to envision the blank, if not hostile, stares that the query would be likely to elicit. Yet this new prospective payment system for Medicare may have great implications for the culture of American medical practice.[2] Furthermore, the Social Security Act Amendments of 1983 (Public Law 98–21) explicitly require the bureaucracy and Congress to explore the "feasibility and desirability of applying the (DRG) payment methodology . . . to payment by all payors for inpatient hospital services." Important distributive issues related to this system need to be debated. Experts representing different groups and ideologies will undoubtedly do so. But it will not be a debate that the populace and media can readily fathom despite its ultimate importance for who gets what medical care, the quality of that care, and its cost.

Third, politics becomes technical to the degree that major decision centers are located in the bureaucracy rather than in the halls of Congress. Technical politics is largely bureaucratic, or executive-branch, politics. The bureaucracy not only plays a major role in shaping the alternatives that the legislative branch considers but also becomes the playing field for the politics of implementation that occurs after a bill becomes law. Elected officials often leave decisions for administrators to resolve during the implementation process. Vague statutes may force civil servants into this role, or the law may explicitly require administrators to make choices affecting who gets what from a health program. For instance, the legislation establishing the DRG payment system for Medicare patients receiving treatment in hospitals leaves many critical issues concerning payment levels to be resolved within the executive branch during the implementation process. The levels of payment established for some 468 different diagnoses will strongly influence the degree to which hospitals face financial pressures to economize and discover more cost-effective modes of medical care. Set one way, these rates would reinforce the status quo; set another, they would probably spawn (for better or worse) considerable change.

In sum, the quest for acceptable ways to constrain costs in the medical sector has come to dominate the policy context in industrialized democracies. This concern with costs is exacerbated by the sense that these societies may well be at the flat of the economist's curve where increased dollar investments in medical care and even preventive health programs will fail to yield impressive gains in health. The politics generated by these concerns is highly technical, featuring marginal adjustment, issues dimly grasped by the great mass of the citizenry, and a shift in major decision making to government bureaucracies.

THE THIRD WORLD: BREAKTHROUGH AND DEMOCRACY

When one turns to the Third World, the policy context changes substantially. Here talk about flat-of-the-curve investments in health as well as technical politics becomes less relevant because in most instances the health problem is a far different one. Life expectancies in these countries tend to be much lower. Infectious disease remains a more potent killer. Malnutrition and unsanitary conditions loom large as sources of disease. These countries tend to spend a much smaller proportion of their GNPs on health care and their medical facilities remain inaccessible to much of the population (World Bank 1975).

In a certain sense, the politics of breakthrough remains a distinct possibility in many of these countries. Given increased resources and the wisdom to build an infrastructure to assure sanitary conditions and adequate food supplies for the populace, governments could realize substantial health gains in relatively short periods of time. Prudent investments in the medical sector could also yield significant health dividends.

The intriguing question in the case of much of the Third World is whether the politics of breakthrough marches hand-in-hand with the rise of authoritarian, albeit egalitarian, states. Achieving and sustaining health gains often requires government to engage in highly coercive practices. Regimes may, for instance, have to place great pressure on the populace to practice birth control in order to sustain health gains. Harsh measures may be required to prevent the squandering of resources on showcase medical facilities in the cities and to encourage a more accessible system of health care that depends less on the acute-care medical model. Can these and similar measures be readily implemented without the imposition of highly coercive egalitarian regimes such as those in Cuba and China? The tension between the politics of breakthrough and the sustenance of democratic procedures goes to the heart of critical policy issues in much of the Third World.

THE ROLE OF APPLIED ANTHROPOLOGY

A straightforward rationale underlies the disproportionate attention given to technical politics in this essay. Anthropologists have long excelled at describing the structures and cultures of communities in less modernized societies. Their potential contribution to discussions of policy in these societies seems evident. By contrast, their ability to inform the policy debates of the more industrialized societies is less widely understood.

Without question, economics ranks as the dominant social science within health policy circles. The application of economic models and methods has undoubtedly contributed valuable insights. Deference to the economic model in formulating health policies can easily become excessive, however. Economists have often been insensitive to the political and organizational issues involved in implementing public policies. In his recent analysis of federal programs to encourage the development of health maintenance organizations, for instance, Brown (1983) masterfully shows how the conceptual baggage of economics with its emphasis on incentives, competition, and the market can lead program advocates at the national level to ignore the complexities of institution building and change at the community level. This neglect often contributes to a substantial gap between expectations and program performance.

A full appreciation of the implications of various policy alternatives requires consideration of the interaction between health programs and communities. This street-level interaction among implementing agents, their clients, and other major actors in the community often spells the difference for whether a policy accomplishes desirable ends (Elmore 1979–80; Lipsky 1980). Applied anthropology can inform us about variations in the structure and culture of the settings where policy ultimately gets delivered; it can dissect the organizational cultures of implementing agents at the street level and the relevance of these cultures for performance (e.g., Friedson 1975). In these and other ways the perspective and methodology of applied anthropology can provide needed leaven for multidisciplinary efforts to develop and assess policy and organizational alternatives in the health arena.

NOTES

1. This distinction draws heavily on Brown (1983:10, 479). See also Thompson (in press).

2. Under the new payment system, the federal government annually and prospectively establishes a fixed price linked to the diagnosis of the Medicare patient. Hospitals receive the same amount from the program for serving a Medicare recipient in a given diagnostic category whether that patient requires a lot or a little care. If a hospital can treat a patient for less money than the government pays for the particular Diagnosis Related Group, it can pocket the difference. Among other things, the system presumably removes any incentive to provide excessive amounts of care once the hospital admits the patient. This system stands in stark contrast to the original Medicare practice of paying hospitals their "reasonable costs" for providing care to the elderly. The old system encouraged hospitals to provide more rather than less service.

Service Delivery, Advocacy, and the Policy Cycle

Michael V. Angrosino and Linda M. Whiteford

This paper rests on the assumption that the most critical issue in health policy *is* health policy. Regardless of the specific problems which are the subjects of decision making, the underlying question is: How is policy *made* (i.e., authored, promoted, implemented, and evaluated)? The question is of particular relevance to the applied social scientist who wishes to contribute meaningfully to the debate on substantive policy issues.

The relevance of this question has been amplified by recent trends in our political system. Among those trends we may discern the general conservative bent of the administration and Congress; increasing skepticism about the value of elements in the great array of "social" programs developed prior to the 1980s; concerns about the size and scope of the federal budget; the shift from categorical to block-grant funding; the emphasis—merely ideological or in practice—on local government support over federal intervention in community service program delivery; and the acceptance of the notions—again, ideologically or actually—of volunteerism and private-sector support for community programs (Champagne and Harpham 1984). Given this emphasis (which is likely to dominate health and human service policy for several years, regardless of the outcome of the 1984 elections), standard assumptions about the "policy process" as derived from the classic policy analysis literature cannot necessarily be taken for granted.

It is therefore the intention of the authors to discuss an alternative to the classic policy analysis model, so as to understand the policy process in light of the new realities of the political system. Using that model, we will analyze two case studies in the emergence of health policy and then consider how the lessons derived from this discussion can be applied by social scientists interested in the development of health policy in the United States.

MODELS OF THE POLICY PROCESS

The Classic Model

Traditional policy analysis has rested on the assumption that policy flows downward, from legislators, administrators, or other elite groups (e.g., Presthus 1974; Thompson 1981:252–82). There is a tendency to treat service agencies simply as implementors of policy insofar as they carry out directives from on high or respond to pressure from some designated service community; but they are almost never viewed as creative partners in the process (Hargrove 1975). The very label "agency" carries with it the connotation of standing in for someone else. There is evidence in the literature to suggest that agency staff often accept their uncreative lot in the delivery of health and human services; the perceived marginality of their position with regard to decision making may be one factor in the development of a "burnout" syndrome among human service workers (Emener 1979).

Proponents of the classic model of policy formation focus on the innovative roles of legislative/executive bodies. They imply that the failure of policy to achieve its stated goals is due to the foot dragging of uncomprehending agency staffs. In the case of public programs, the latter may form a kind of permanent bureaucracy that goes on and on even as the creative planners come and go. Having no stake in the game of shifting policy directives, agencies can thus easily be perceived as mere cogs in the wheels of the policy process.

With the new emphasis on local initiatives, however, it seems clear that if policy is to continue to evolve, then those most directly involved in service delivery will have to take a more active role. The case studies in this paper treat of two instances in which policy was developed on the initiative of either a service agency or a local-level advocacy group. One case, that of Child Watch, reflects conditions in the post-1980 political arena. The other, that of the Human Development Center, predates that watershed. A comparison of the two cases should therefore be instructive as we develop an alternative to the classic model of policy analysis.

A Critique of the Classic Model

Public policy has been defined as "whatever governments choose to do or not to do" (Dye 1972:1). In other words, the making of policy requires a set of options from which a decision maker must select a course of action. The task of traditional policy analysis was to identify and clarify those options. While some social scientists have been able to become decision makers themselves, as in C. Wright Mills's "philosopher king" analogy, most anthropologists interested in policy have played Mills's role of "adviser to the king" (1950:179–81). They have seen themselves as "knowledge transfer specialists" (Hobbs 1979) who ransack the scholarly literature on a given issue, translate it into everyday English, and present a set of clear-cut recommendations to decision makers. This task is a worthy one, but it seems to have caused us to lose sight of some basic theoretical guideposts from our own discipline.

The "knowledge transfer" approach has apparently led us to think of policy as a simple input-output process, such as one finds in the rationalist school of political science theory (Finsterbusch and Motz 1980:23–39; Frohock 1979). The problem with this model from an anthropological perspective is that it neglects to place policy in its widest social and cultural context, for it sees policy as a process and an end in itself. Policy may be, in Dye's terms, a decision; and that decision may be based on the clarifying analyses of social scientists. But decision makers are part of a social network, as are the policy analysts. Because their decisions may affect society at large, there is at least the possibility that the policy decision may have a stone-in-pond effect, stirring up as many implications for new ideas, or requirements for problems to be solved, as it does definitive solutions. Those being decided for should logically be seen as offering their own input into decision making, in the form of their response to policy. Even outright resistance should be seen not as a dead end, but as a creative response, insofar as it stimulates a reformulation of policy. Moreover, because policy does not begin with reasoned input and end with a rational decision, the possibility exists that the locus of decision making will move through a social network with each succeeding decision.

For example, in 1946 Congress passed the Mental Health Act, which recognized some basic service needs of that era by providing for psychiatric and mental health research (Ozarin 1982). It also created a centralized administrative agency, the National Institute of Mental Health (NIMH), to implement the guidelines for training and research. But the NIMH, by faithfully implementing the mandate for training and research, spawned a new generation of mental health professionals whose concerns were not with institutional psychiatry, but with community-based treatment. That shift in emphasis in service delivery was not entirely unintended on the part of the framers of the act, but neither was it a primary goal. The NIMH was set up to administer a few specific programs; but by using its discretion about whom to fund, and for what projects, NIMH in effect replaced Congress as the primary decision maker with regard to mental health policy. (The number of anthropologists whose fieldwork was supported by NIMH over the years is testimony to the degree to which this agency broadened and transformed its original mandate.)

The standard model of legislation leading to the creation of an agency to implement policy must certainly be broadened to include the evolution of the agency's own perception of its role and scope. It is, in this case, a fairly safe assumption that the rise of a citizens' advocacy movement in mental health was stimulated by the pro-outpatient outlook fostered by NIMH in the 1950s, and that that movement—rather than "policy analysis research" in the congressional staffs—impelled the president to appoint the Joint Commission on Mental Health and Illness in 1961. It was from that commission's investigations that the Community Mental Health Centers Act of 1963 sprang, and with it the modern "revolution" in mental health practice (Wagenfeld and Jacobs 1982).

The Cyclic Model: An Alternative to the Classic Model

A more congenial model for understanding the ever-expanding evolutionary sequence is that represented by the *policy cycle* approach (May and Wildavsky 1978). Analysts in this school have identified eleven steps that move a mere "good idea" to the status of implemented policy. These steps may be summarized as follows (Jones 1984:27–28):

1. *Perception/definition.* What is the specific problem which needs to be addressed? Do I have a good idea as to how it should be addressed?

2. *Aggregation*. Can I convince some other people that my idea is a good one?
3. *Organization*. Can I form this group of concerned citizens into a body that can be effectively mobilized for action?
4. *Representation*. Does our organization have access to decision makers? If not, how can such access be obtained and maintained?
5. *Agenda-setting*. How can we convince the decision makers that the issue is one deserving of priority attention?
6. *Formulation*. Can workable, feasible solutions be devised?
7. *Legitimization*. Can the solution of choice be supported by all the people needed to make it work?
8. *Budgeting*. Can adequate funding be allocated to support this solution?
9. *Implementation*. Can an appropriate agency be set up to carry out this mandate?
10. *Evaluation*. Is the agency achieving its stated goals? Do gaps in service still exist? Why? Are they amenable to solution?
11. *Adjustment*. Can the program be modified so as to deal with perceived gaps? Is additional programming necessary?

It is clear, in reviewing this model, that the making of decisions is only one small part of a much larger process, a process involving many more actors than simply the analyst and the decision maker. Moreover, it is in the nature of this process to be cyclical. Policy does not stop with implementation, for the evaluation of implemented programs generates new information about unanticipated consequences which may require new policy solutions in the future (see table 1).

The Cyclic Model: An Anthropological Perspective

What is striking about this cyclical model is its harmony with very traditional anthropological theory, specifically Malinowskian functionalism as represented in *A Scientific Theory of Culture* (1944). It will be remembered that Malinowski's premise was that all human beings come equipped with basic needs which he did not precisely label, but which may be grouped under the rubric "nurturance." These needs are a consequence of the biological fact that human infants are

Table 1

Comparison of Alternative Policy Models

Traditional Model	Revisionist/Activist Model
Policy flows downward from legislators, administrators, etc. Agencies seen as implementers of policy Agencies not seen as creative in the policy process Agency seen as bureaucratic quagmire Community advocates seen as making suggestions to primary decision makers	Policy generated from the community level, based on locally perceived need Agencies seen as creative identifiers of policy needs Agencies seen as legitimate repository of justification of client need Agencies seen as implementors and evaluators of services

born in a helpless condition. Their need for nurturance is the genesis of human social systems, for every society must create a set of "primary institutions" to satisfy these basic needs.

However, Malinowski recognized that no society is composed simply of primary institutions, for the latter create unintended problems of their own. Institutions which develop to meet these newly discerned needs are known as "secondary institutions." The process of need generation is not a static one (despite the charges so often levelled indiscriminately at all the functionalists), for institutions have the capacity to create as many new problems as they solve old ones; a living society is continuously in the process of generating needs. To put this concept somewhat differently, the culture engenders "striving sentiments," and a healthy society will evolve to help people achieve those perceived needs by modifying old institutions or even generating new ones (Leighton 1959:395–420).

Malinowski's functionalism, therefore, is a matter of seeing beyond the need-satisfaction of any part of the social system in order to understand the way in which the generation of needs and the evolution of institutions form a complex whole. Society is thus a large, functionally integrated feedback loop, with a culture and value system to give meaning to that integration. The function of the whole is to permit the continuing adaptation of the society to its environment—an environment which it helps modify, or even create.

Given Malinowski's and Leighton's insights into the processes of functional adaptation of the society as a whole, it becomes clearer that the policy cycle is itself part of a social institution of governance which modifies and even helps create the social environment and which aids in the adaptation of the community at large, at least in the short run. If that is the case, it may be possible to move beyond the model of analyst-and-decision-maker to an understanding of policy as a social process.

One of the relatively few anthropologists to have approached issues of how a modern society organizes to administer policy is A. F. C. Wallace, who has pointed out that modern industrial societies are characterized by the presence of "administrative structures" composed of three social groups: owners (or those under whose auspices work is done); target populations or clienteles; and administrative organizations themselves (1971:1–2). The latter are defined as the "action groups" in this set, and they are "responsible *for* the clientele and responsible *to* the owners" (1971:2). The "action group" is the vehicle by which "owners" (such as the government) achieve their impact on the clientele. According to Wallace, there is a tendency, as societies evolve toward greater complexity, for administrative structures to survive by a process of "insulation," the adaptation of an ethical principle that seeks to eliminate as far as possible any personal factor in administration. The agency is supposed to be a value-neutral carrier out of policy (1971:5).

However, Wallace believes that it is inherent in the nature of administrative structures to be engaged in an almost constant process of "aging and reorganization," a process composed of incremental changes in structures analogous to the processes of his more famous revitalization model. This gradual process is necessitated by the tendency in administrative structures toward "corruption," by which he means "a kind of emotional or social entropy" (1971:7). On a more positive note, however, administrative structures also need to "respond to changes in the demands made on them by their owners or by their target/clientele populations" (1971:8).

Administrative structures, despite their tendency toward insulation and corruption, are part of a self-correcting and adaptable system. Our only point of departure from Wallace's view is in the attempt to demonstrate that the impetus for change can arise from *within* the agency (or administrative structure) or from advocates from the client community if they mobilize in certain ways. But what are the conditions under which such groups may take up a creative role? Case studies which demonstrate the assumption of an activist role on the part of structures not usually thought of as creative partners in the traditional model will illustrate this process.

TWO CASE STUDIES: HOW LOCAL STRUCTURES BECOME CREATIVE PARTNERS IN THE POLICY CYCLE

Case 1: The Human Development Center

The Human Development Center (HDC) is a program that provides community-based treatment for clients with the dual diagnosis of (mild or moderate) mental retardation and emotional disturbance; many of the clients have also been in trouble with the law and have been adjudicated to the HDC in lieu of prison or a state institution. The program serves approximately twenty males at a time. There is, as of this writing, a very wide client age range (fourteen through forty-three), although the focus is on those between the ages of eighteen and twenty-five. Clients live in three strictly supervised group homes in a small town approximately twenty miles from downtown Tampa, and during the day they attend the Sunrise Skills Center, located in the city of Tampa, where they learn vocational and academic skills. The programs are structured along behavior modification lines with graded groups, a point system, and token economy (Creer and Christian 1976:ch. 7; Drash, Stoffel, and Murdock 1983; Schwartz 1973). Clients move up from "group 1," progressively acquiring more skills, responsibilities, and privileges. Successful clients are placed in an independent living program with minimal staff supervision. One innovation of particular interest is the HDC's use of the peer group in its behavior modification system. All resident clients have the right to vote on whether another client is ready to "move up." They also form a kind of appeals court if a client is to be "busted" to a lower group by the staff for some infraction of the rules. These peer groups meet regularly both at the group homes and at the Skills Center, and have an important part in the process of developing a sense of independence and responsibility in the clients.

The HDC was the first program in the state of Florida designed to serve this dually diagnosed clientele. Its success has made it something of a model program. However, a review of the history of HDC will demonstrate that it was not an "agent" of state policy, but rather a creative initiator of policy.

HDC began in 1975 under the auspices of the local Association for Retarded Citizens (ARC). ARCs are advocacy groups, usually composed of parents or guardians of retarded persons, plus professionals in the field of mental retardation, and they have had a significant impact on the development of an enlightened public consciousness about mental retardation (Holland 1980). The ARC serving the Tampa area was particularly vigorous in the 1970s because its chairperson happened to be a member of the state legislature, a gentleman who had staked out the area of health and human services as his particular concern. He saw to it that the ARC expanded into the field of direct services, and one of its new programs was to be the HDC, designed to serve delinquent retarded teenagers. (The original plan was for both boys and girls to be served, but as the first clients to be admitted were males, and since no funds were forthcoming to establish separate domiciliary facilities for females, the program had an all-male clientele, a situation which has continued.) We can therefore see that the recognition of service needs in this case occurred as a result of the close working relationship between a citizen advocacy group and an influential legislator. Out of that partnership there arose a new direction of policy: a newly defined clientele in need of services, and a newly defined role of service provision for what had hitherto been a strictly advocacy organization. The HDC thus first played a classic role of agent of others' policy initiatives.

HDC operated under ARC auspices for three years, by which time three members of the staff had come to the realization that the program that had been hoped for was being left by the wayside by precisely those who had inspired it. The ARC as a whole never liked its service delivery role, and was already taking steps to divest itself of all but its advocacy and community education functions. The state government, having set up the program, was unwilling to foster it and seemed willing to let it languish with insufficient funding. The stereotypical response to this frustration has been staff burnout. In this case, however, the three staff members decided to fight for what they believed in, and arranged a separation from the ARC; the HDC was born as an independent, nonprofit organization under separate contract to the state.

The new HDC had two basic tasks: to convince the state that its client population was a significant one (for in the long run it would be more cost-efficient to train the young men for independent living in the community than to keep them in the state's institutional care for the rest of their lives); and, of course, to convince the state to come up with adequate funding. The task was made all the more difficult by the fact that the local representative of the state's Department of Health and Rehabilitative Services (HRS) was impatient with the notion of "rehabilitation," his health care model being medical/treatment in orientation rather than developmental. Moreover, the original HDC staffers, for reasons of personality and political ideology, were not inclined to be compliant bureaucrats, and they refused to allow their program to die by inches like good "agents" should.

The confrontation between a small program serving a clientele most people would prefer to ignore on the one hand, and the state health department on the other would hardly have captured the public's fancy in such a way as to effect a major change in policy were it not for the fact that at the same time the state was pinching pennies with HDC, it was supporting a program purporting to serve the same clientele—at a cheaper rate. This program was run by members of a religious sect with authoritarian tendencies; corporal punishment was their preferred means of behavior modification. Unlike the HDC, which demanded a considerable budget to support a well-trained staff and extensive programs of vocational and academic training, this other program seemed relatively inexpensive to the state, which indicated its intention to decline to renew its contract with HDC and to move the HDC clients to the other program.

With the aid of a sympathetic local reporter, the HDC staffers produced evidence of the physical abuse practiced at the other center, as well as of certain bookkeeping irregularities. The story broke in the press that the state was letting a legitimate program die for lack of funds while supporting a group of untrained religious zealots to the tune of $500,000 per year. There was consequent public outrage not only about the abuse of the poor, helpless clients, but also about the administrative issue of the state having no functional means of monitoring services delivered in its name.

Practicing "confrontation politics," the HDC staff took its clients to the state capital where they camped out in the halls of the legislature. This spectacle inspired the legislators to direct HRS to sign a contract with HDC at a "reasonable rate." The HRS complied, but with notable bad grace. There was a month lapse, during which time the staff voluntarily worked without pay—pay which has never been reimbursed. There have been problems over the years with HRS deliberately withholding clients from HDC, but the basic relationship has been stabilized.

It is now accepted state practice to monitor all its vendors (i.e., private organizations that deliver community-based services to state clients under contract) for compliance with fiscal regulations as well as for reasonable client outcomes. (The larger issues of quality assurance in a vendor system of community services are treated comparatively in Angrosino 1981.)

From this brief review, we can see that two very significant elements in current state policy (specifically for mentally retarded clients, but easily extended to the mental health system as a whole) have been established, not by the traditional actors (the state government—legislative and executive) but by the humble agents of policy, working in conjunction with local advocates. These two elements are as follows:

1. It is both proper and feasible to set up service programs for dually diagnosed clients. State policy has traditionally relied on a criterion of unitary diagnosis, such that mentally retarded clients and emotionally disturbed clients are reasonably well served; but clients with both problems (not to mention other complicating factors, such as physical handicaps or involvement in the juvenile justice system) have been shut out. The usual response is the designation of a "primary diagnosis," which means that a caseworker will arbitrarily decide which of the problems is of greater importance, such that the client can at least be served in one system.

2. The state has a moral as well as a political responsibility to the public to assure that programs funded to serve its clients are in fact upholding acceptable standards of fiscal practice and therapeutic regimen.

The agency was able to establish these principles, despite the opposition (or, at best, the passive neutrality) of both the legislature and the organized advocacy community for two main reasons. On one hand, the innovations of the HDC were part of a process of adaptive radiation, as the HDC strategy was to move itself into an unoccupied niche. No other agency served such clients (who had, in fact, been legislated out of existence by the "unitary diagnosis" criterion); remember that the ARC plan was to serve "delinquent" retarded teenagers, not necessarily those with the specific problems grouped under the title "emotional disturbance." As a result, no entrenched interests were directly challenged. There was certainly the obstacle of tradition: the feeling that since such a population had never been served, then it could never be possible to serve them. But that feeling is quite different from one that might be expressed by an entrenched bureaucracy which felt its own turf to be directly threatened. In effect, the HDC, by following its own head, proved that it *could* be done and, in so doing, started people thinking about the benefits (economic and social) of doing it. "Why didn't anyone think of this before?" can become a potent cry that pushes an issue onto the decision maker's agenda. The state responded primarily by allocating funds to serve this population, although the HRS at first chose to direct those funds to an agency other than the one that had raised the issue. The new service orientation was established as a priority by the power of the state's budget, but the HDC was in danger of being cut off because it had dared to step out of its accepted role.

On the other hand, the independence of the HDC meant that it was not part of the bureaucratic establishment, and so had nothing to lose by taking its case to "the streets" rather than "working through channels." Since it had no stake in the structure, the HDC could mobilize the press and civil liberties attorneys, and through them the public at large. That the state had the right to allocate funds for a desirable service to any vendor it chose was not the issue. What was at issue was whether, once having allocated such monies, the state did not have an obligation to see that the taxpayers' dollars were being wisely spent. This is a question no one inside the structure could afford to ask, for who could tell where the eye of scrutiny would fall? The HDC had, in the structural sense, nothing to lose by taking a moral stance on the issue. It knew it was delivering good service and anyway was going to go out of business if *no* state accountability system were established. Because of the dramatic nature of the confrontation—which HDC orchestrated—it forced the state to accept its principles. In demonstrating their own principled nature by working for nothing when necessary, the staff members publicly demonstrated their moral superiority.

The principles upheld by HDC thus became state policy and went through the stages of the cycle outlined above, but with the crucial difference that the innovation began with the agency set up to implement an older policy in which inconsistencies had been discerned.

Discussion of Case 1

An organization can have a creative part in the policy cycle by making the powers that be more aware of unmet needs that can feasibly be dealt with, and by depicting itself as sufficiently outside the system to engage in a meaningful critique of that system—and yet, of course, not so far outside that it seems just a gadfly. The state was made to understand that it needed HDC, with all its obstreperous antics, more than the HDC needed the state, once a demand had been identified for service to a client population that could not be served by any other reputable agency. The HDC was able to take the higher ground: the staff had no *personal* stake in the outcome of the confrontation—it was the welfare of the clients (and, by extension, all the helpless wards of the state) that became the public issue.

The question must certainly arise: Now that the HDC is an established program with an excellent community reputation and reasonably amicable relations with the state, has it been co-opted? Is it too closely identified with a certain client population ever to engage in further "adaptive radiation"? Is it too much a part of the system to ever again be willing or able to present itself as a moral alternative to state policy? As of this writing, it seems as if HDC is determined to keep its activist role alive, despite the pressure to find a comfortable niche in the system. It has taken two steps in that direction:

1. In the past year, the staff has given voice to a conclusion that might have been unthinkable just a few years ago: Not all clients are capable of "graduation." For some, the severity of the behavioral problems is such that it is unrealistic to expect them to become independent members of the community, although they can still lead pro-

ductive lives under close supervision. The clients sense the frustration of learning skills but never being able to graduate, and hence the benefits of the program are vitiated. Current policy posits an option: the institution, or independent living in the community. HDC is now in the process of defining a third alternative: the creation of a special group home in the community (i.e., not on the same campus with the basic group homes) with a degree of supervision intermediate between the group homes and the independent apartment program. Students with irremediable behavior problems could successfully "graduate" to this new kind of home setting, without the stigma attached to perennial failures to attain independent living status. Hence, HDC staff are on the cutting edge again by defining new service options, not only for their own existing clients, but also for those referred directly into this new intermediate group home program from other programs around the state. In other words, the Malinowskian equation of one solution generating new needs that require new solutions has been operative.

2. The staff itself has called for—and has called into existence—a strong, independent board of trustees. Not just a standard "letterhead" board of community worthies, the HDC board is composed of people with an active interest in the clients and the rehabilitation program. The board is involved in long-range planning and has direct oversight in areas of client services, physical plant, financial management, and community awareness. Because the board members are, by and large, persons with their own reputations in the community and not beholden to HRS, the board has become a force for maintaining the in-the-system-but-not-of-it status of HDC. The particular nature of the board makes it possible for the HDC to maintain its reputation as a critic and rethinker of HRS policy, even while the program itself operates comfortably within the framework of the HRS system. In sum, it was the agency which created the board, to serve its own needs (i.e., to play the part of moral arbiter which the staff members, now entered into a working partnership with HRS, could no longer comfortably perform); it mobilized the community to serve those needs, rather than vice versa.

Case 2: Child Watch

Child Watch was a local fact-finding and advocacy project organized in response to President Reagan's budget reductions. The project was organized by the Children's Defense Fund (CDF), a Washington, D.C.–based advocacy and lobbying group. In Tampa the project was composed of a coalition of voluntary public service groups. The task of Child Watch was to trace how the loss of federal monies had a local impact on the delivery of social services, particularly those in the area of health care delivery to children.

"Since 1980, children have come first in budget sacrifice. They lost one of every ten dollars previously provided them by their national government for critical preventive children's and family support programs" (Children's Defense Fund 1984:15). "Children also have been the first victims of poverty. More than 3.1 million children, 3,000 a day, have fallen into poverty since 1979. Their thirty-one percent poverty increase is the sharpest rise in child poverty since poverty statistics have been collected. Less than one-third of these new poor children will be lifted from poverty by economic recovery alone" (Children's Defense Fund 1984:17).

The lack of a clearly articulated national child health policy opened the way for the president to propose $11 billion in cuts in programs crucial to children's well-being in 1982; the following year he further proposed an additional cut of $9 billion in those programs. In fiscal year 1984 the administration asked that more than $3.5 billion be additionally cut from those programs, and in fiscal 1985 an additional $3 billion in cuts is sought.

The lack of a national child health policy made such fiscal restructuring possible; it also provided the impetus for advocacy and lobbying activities resulting in local and national policy changes. The resultant developments in child health policies were generated from outside the traditional policy-creation channels. The following case study is an example of the policy cycle as a social process. Child Watch provides an opportunity to trace the development of health policy from its inception as a response to severe fiscal budget reductions, through local advocacy activity and centralized nationwide research, to its contribution to the Children's Survival Bill (H.R. 1603, S. 572) being introduced in the U.S. Congress in the spring of 1984.

In order to understand policy development as a social process, it is important to review briefly some of the history and structure of child health care policy in the United States. In 1912, President Theodore Roosevelt created the federal Children's Bureau in an effort to improve health care for mothers and children. In 1921 Congress passed the

Sheppard-Towner Maternity Act to promote the "welfare and hygiene of maternity and infancy" (Children's Defense Fund 1984:43) by providing federal funding to help states in that effort. The programs incorporated in the Sheppard-Towner Maternity Act later (1935) became the basis of the Title V Maternal and Child Health Program. In 1935 Congress enacted the Aid to Dependent Children (ADC) Program as part of the Social Security Act; ADC was designed to provide families in which one parent was dead or missing with financial support to raise the children. The cost of the program was shared between state and federal budgets. In 1950 Congress passed the Social Security Act Amendments which specifically created a medical assistance program providing matching federal funds for health care services purchased for ADC children. In the fifteen years between 1950 and 1965, the federal government strengthened this program of medical assistance, which in 1965 became the Medicaid Program. An important aspect of the historical development of child welfare legislation is that it shows the development and institution of a set of attitudes, values, and goals, all of which (though covertly) have been challenged by the present administration.

Initially, the urgency to analyze the data generated by Child Watch was very real: the data were needed to document the effect of loss of services and to present arguments against further reductions in federal aid for children's health care costs. The research findings had to be available for analysis and presentation before the next fiscal budget was presented to Congress. Once that early information was sent to Washington, it became obvious that the data served to raise questions requiring continued research. After two phases of the research were completed, the evaluation and public presentation of that information generated local concern over the consequences of loss of federal monies on the welfare of children in the community. Congruent with the third phase of research, a local public awareness and education campaign was undertaken in conjunction with lobbying efforts on behalf of changes in health care policy.

Before we describe in more detail the activities that went into this project and the implications thereof for policymaking, let us point out how these activities exemplify the cyclical process of policy creation. Policy development viewed from the procedural orientation incorporates the following elements: the identification and analysis of a problem or a problematic situation; the involvement of a decision maker recommending changes in policy; and the implementation of those policy recommendations. Once the recommended changes have occurred, evaluation of those changes and the consequences of those changes are analyzed in light of new problems and new policy solutions. This model closely approximates the activities occurring during the operation of Child Watch.

Child Watch came about as a result of a need to document changes in health status as a response to changes in health policy. While human service professionals and others could both anticipate and imagine the effects of loss of federal revenues on local programs to a disadvantaged and voiceless population, imagination could not provide the kind of quantifiable data that were needed. What was needed was statistical evidence gathered locally during the time that the reductions were being translated into programmatic changes. Responding to this situation, impetus from a national organization provided the mechanism by which local groups began to gather data addressing the question. That mechanism took the form of a standardized series of questions to be asked of specific categories of people in health and human services. Two hundred fifty interviews were conducted in an eighteen-month period. Four topical areas were identified as programs significant to the welfare of children and at the same time heavily dependent upon federal support: child health, child welfare, day care, and aid to families with dependent children. Within each topical area, interviews were conducted with program administrators and policymakers, providers, advocates, and clients of these programs.

Certain decisions were made at CDF that structured the local project. One of those decisions was that local researchers were to focus on the policymakers, those who carry out the policies, and those whose lives were being affected by those policies. The relationships among federal, state, and local policymakers were made an explicit part of the research design. The social process of decision making, implementation, and evaluation was, in part, captured by the project as it measured program and policy changes by interviewing the same people about the same programs at three-month intervals.

Child Watch information had input into policy decisions in several ways. First, information was sent to Washington. There, the staff of the CDF broke it down and analyzed it. The information was collected with the knowledge that it would be used both locally and nationally. With that knowledge in mind, we sought information on the history of services, changes in programs over the last several years, and other information that would provide a context in which to understand the potential, as well as the real, impact of the changes taking place. Knowledge of the intended use of the findings made it possible to collect data that would make that information valuable in policy decisions.

The results of Child Watch were shared with a number of people and organizations. Through CDF the information was delivered as testimony at the U.S. Senate Hearings, Subcommittee on Nutrition of the Committee on Agriculture, Nutrition, and Forestry. State as well as federal legislators were informed of the project's findings. Television, radio, and newspaper interviews were given; brief summaries were supplied to local newspapers and neighborhood newsletters. During the project a grassroots coalition of groups was created. Each of these groups was mailed both updates of the findings as the research progressed, and an analysis of the final conclusions of the research project. CDF also sent out a nationwide newsletter focusing on the Child Watch results. This newsletter was sent to each project approximately every three months. The newsletter contained findings of importance selected from all the Child Watch projects around the nation, thereby providing access to comparative data.

On the basis of the information produced, the Child Watch coalition chose to take an active role in the development of health care policy for children of the poor. This decision was facilitated, in part, by providing documentation of need, as well as structured, programmatic recommendations to policymakers. Channeling Child Watch information to policymakers occurred in two ways: vertically from the local project to CDF in Washington, and from there to members of Congress; and horizontally between various projects via the CDF newsletter. Information moved from the local project to state and local legislators, and to the supporting organizations as well as to the local public.

Many of the recommendations made by Child Watch revolved around the issue of child health care and the lack of access to care for children of the indigent. (At the time of the initial research, no local private practice pediatrician would see a Medicaid child in his or her office.) As a direct result of this project, two pediatricians and several nurses have set up free clinics three times a year to treat children of migrant farm workers, children who otherwise would have been without medical care. At the same time, Child Watch was able to provide documentation of the inadequacy of child health policy at a time when there was a local initiative to create both a children's hospital and a freestanding children's clinic (especially designed to care for poor children). Health care policy that explicitly focused on the provision of health care to children of the poor was made a specific focus of the founding philosophy for the new health care institutions. The children's hospital and the clinic are planned for the near future. By focusing attention on a particular problem and by providing legitimization of that problem through documentation, Child Watch moved actively into the policy process.

Discussion of Case 2

Policy implications of this research can be seen at several different levels. First is a redefinition of a particular population. Children of the poor, and, more recently, the newly enlarged category of children of the working poor, were reconceptualized as a category of people at risk. In the past, they were easily ignored because they had little power within the political system. Federal programs designed to care for children have been perceived as causing deficits in the budget; in truth, those very programs are deficit containers if they protect and prepare children for self-sufficiency. Child Watch, by focusing attention on this population, its unmet needs, and the potential social and economic costs associated with lack of preventive health care, highlighted the need for specific policy development on these children's behalf.

This particular population (sick children of indigent parents) is a category caught between publicly expressed beliefs in the welfare of all children and the private support of a fiscally conservative government. As local agencies responded to the Child Watch research, an advocacy coalition recognizing this category of children was created. In a sense, the budget cuts provided the opportunity for legitimization of this at-risk population. While the plight of poor children, especially in the area of health care, was very real before the budget cuts, those reductions so exacerbated an already intolerable situation as to almost "force" policy to be written and legislation to be created to protect children.

The second way in which health policy was influenced, and has the potential for continued influence, is through the coalition of agencies and individuals drawn together in this effort. Child Watch served as a central research and advocacy body which contacted, and was contacted by, individuals concerned about the health of children. Originally, people were contacted to work on the project, or to provide information and expertise in the development of a data base. Many of these people became sponsors of Child Watch. Sponsors were people with whom we shared our findings, who lent support and often credibility to our public statements. They formed a loose network, tied by their interest and commitment to the topic. Others joined the coalition because of their professional involvement in child health. Administrators, state and regional elected representatives, and others who were interviewed repeatedly in the process of the research joined the network and took their professional involvement another step beyond vocation to advocacy. In this way, Child Watch provided an avenue, a mechanism, to draw people together without binding them in a structural way. The resulting policy implications of such a coalition were powerful and immediate. Because of the reasons people were drawn together, the lack of structural constraints, and their own personal and professional power in the community, changes became possible that otherwise would not have been imaginable.

Child Watch is but one example of how policy can develop outside the traditional channels: it demonstrates how something that is structured as a research-based coalition can become an advocate, help redefine the perception of a category of people, and provide a mechanism to aid adaptation of the community at large. Because of its structure, Child Watch was able to respond to issues in the national political arena as they were translated into health care systems on the local level. Its local application, particularly in the area of health policy, reflected the concern, commitment, and action of individuals and, as such, the social process of policy development and implementation. The next phase of Child Watch incorporates monitoring and evaluating new services and the consequences of the present policy decisions. One might well anticipate that the analysis of new services and policy solutions will engender identification of new problems, thus continuing the cyclical process of policy development.

CONCLUSION

The two case studies presented here clearly demonstrate how service and advocacy agencies can function as creative initiators of policy. Each case is a description of the development of policy as a social process. It is important to note the similarities shared by the HDC and Child Watch, both in their structures and in the type of client they serve (see table 2). In each case, the client population could be said to be dually disadvantaged. In the case of HDC, the clients were mentally retarded and emotionally disturbed. In the case of Child Watch, the clients were poor and children, both characteristics that traditionally deny them access to power. Both HDC and Child Watch clients were, until recently, unrecognized or were denied recognition as legitimately

Table 2
Similarities Between HDC and Child Watch

Clients	Structure
Dually disadvantaged	Input to policy from outside format
Unrecognized by general public	channels
Legitimacy of need denied at policy level	Members of HDC and Child Watch recognized as "authorities" in
Community-based population	the community but not members
Noninstitutionalized population	of bureaucracy
Outpatient treatment regimens	Provided mechanism for criticism of
Parents or guardians unable to provide for them	service without jeopardizing individuals' jobs
Clients unable to advocate their own rights	Filled a void in extant services or advocacy
	Created a public sentiment for client population
	Responsed to local needs
	Developed extralocal policy issues reflective of national interest

"needy" populations. The client populations were community-based, as opposed to institutionally housed. For both populations—mentally retarded adults and economically deprived children—their needs for survival exceeded their parents/guardians' abilities to provide for them. It is this discrepancy between needs and abilities that makes clients of them. As a population, their inability to speak as their own advocates places them in a position of dependence on others who can present their case in public.

The greatest structural similarity between HDC and Child Watch is in their both being external to extant bureaucracies, and yet having credibility in the eyes of those very bureaucrats. In both cases, the agencies provided a mechanism by which people could channel criticism of the bureaucratic structure into the open without either jeopardizing their jobs or creating internecine antagonism. The two case studies demonstrate how policy can be influenced from the middle level and from the outside; they also show how such outside organizations can fill voids left by institutional superstructures.

The process being described in this paper is not restricted to the two case studies. The two cases encompass many variations. One case has been in existence for a number of years, while the other has only recently begun. One has a paid staff, and the other is strictly volunteer. One began from a grassroots initiative, while the other developed in response to a need perceived in Washington. Yet between them they exemplify both the social process of policy development and the role an anthropologist can play in it.

Anthropologists working in service agencies are particularly well suited to having an impact on policy decisions because of their methodological and conceptual skills. In the two cases presented here, anthropologists were able to respond to local needs by gathering data and conceptualizing problems reflective of issues being focused on at a larger scale. The result was a legitimization of a particular population as one of need and deserving of attention. The process was that of using the anthropologist as a credible outsider to distill real data out of the political and social "noise" and to formulate programmatic policy recommendations based on that information. In the instance of Child Watch, once the population was recognized as legitimate, and its problems as valid, local groups began to be the population's advocates. On the national level, a bill was introduced into Congress to protect the rights of children. Locally, pediatricians and others were made aware of and developed a concern for the lack of medical care available to poor children, and they began to design both a freestanding outpatient clinic (to provide services at no cost to the indigent) and a children's hospital, a portion of whose beds are to be reserved for the needy. In the case of HDC, the initial identification of a dually diagnosed, legitimate service population was followed by the identification of new services that could best serve the needs of that population; these service innovations were underscored by HDC's ability to get the state to recognize and systematize a process for monitoring community-based services delivered in its name.

In sum, the model suggested here sees policy as part of a complex feedback process, with solutions to one problem raising new issues to be solved by new solutions—new solutions, which might be developed by players in the policy cycle, other than those posited in the classic policy analytic literature. In the cases presented here, the creative change agents were located in programs set up to implement older policies; but perceiving new needs, and in a position to act on their own initiatives, they both stimulated important policy shifts. Given the new orientation toward local initiatives, the fact that both of these programs effectuated change in policy without first seeking the approval of the relevant central authority should be an object lesson to applied social scientists; one can have an impact on policy development at the sometimes more accessible middle level of service provision and advocacy without having to be an advisor to the "king."

The applied social scientist can serve to clarify the policy process for agency staff so that they become more aware of their potentially creative role. He or she can also conduct research that results in a reconceptualization of a given service population so as to legitimize change in the service delivery system. By working with an agency newly armed with a positive identity resulting from its active role in policy development, the applied social scientist can work within the new realities of the political system and become an effective player in the policy cycle, combining in the process the roles of researcher and advocate.

Health Care and Bureaucratic Reforms: Clinical and Cultural Paradigms of Care in an Urban-Ethnic Setting

Andrew J. Gordon

Robert Alford's book *Health Care Politics* examines attempted reforms in New York City's health care system. This work focuses on what Alford describes as bureaucratic reforms, those designed to improve the access and efficiency of health care services. Neither his conclusions nor his Marxist-oriented analysis are, today, altogether innovative or surprising. He finds political and economic centers of power holding back true reforms. In his language, the structurally dominant sectors, or those aspiring to be so, organize health care to shore up their own power and wealth, and thereby they deny care to the repressed structures, basically the poor and those without the ability to pay for their health care. *Health Care Politics* describes the expression of political and economic self-interest of hospital administrators, physicians, and private and public organizations who ostensibly attempted to reform the health care system. A great contribution of Alford's book lies in its critical approach to health care reform, an approach disclosing those who really benefit from reforms. The approach itself goes far to inspire other inquiries into reform.

Here I will reflect on field work in a New England Hispanic community (see Gordon 1978, 1979, 1981a and b, n.d.).[1] I examined drinking problems, their treatment, and the inability of the health care reforms to address the problems.

The case in point also highlights insufficiencies in health care delivery as well as problems in reforms to urban-ethnic groups. Alcoholism and its treatment brings larger problems into sharper focus because it reveals how the health care system is limited in addressing the prevention or early treatment of many chronic diseases that are largely the outcome of life-style: many cancers, cardiovascular diseases, and mental health problems. Thus, my point is that even if bureaucratic reforms can fairly distribute care, we have to question if the care itself is in the best interest of the recipients, the patients. Or, alternatively stated, does health care attack the roots of the problem or wait for the full-blown disorder to develop before proceeding with medical care?

Alford is right in that bureaucratic reforms are made into a sham. But, from a cultural perspective, Alford's point of view perhaps misses some salient points. It assumes health care is without its own cultural and behavioral paradigm that would preclude health care functioning in the patient's best interest.

As will be discussed in this paper, this paradigm of health care and medicine may be described in terms of the reliance on experts and specialists as opposed to generalist care, the focus on curing pressing problems as opposed to anticipating possible ones, the subjective experience of having one's problem and discomfort converted into a clinical history, and, finally, the inclination to encapsulate care in the clinical setting as opposed to disseminating care throughout the community. Additionally, this paper will discuss cultural resources for resolving alcoholism problems independently of the health care system. These resources suggest broader strategies for dealing with health problems intimately related to life-style.

Examining alcoholism services in the last decade is particularly interesting because this short history reveals how the health care system adapted a problem that had been addressed behaviorally in terms of social codes and cultural models of treatment—or indigenous treatment—and converted it into a medical issue. Furthermore, the approach to alcoholism, much of which evolved as a result of reforms in the health care system, identifies the influences of medicine on attempts to innovate and to reform health care. In this paper, I will first describe the cultural or indigenous approaches to the alcoholism problem that are pursued by the Hispanic population. Then I move on to discuss the reforms and their fate in the Hispanic community. What I will attempt to show is that not only does the Hispanic community not receive its just share of services, but that even if services were fairly distributed, a whole different approach to care would need to be formulated.

The Setting

Alcoholism and its treatment will be examined in a population of 15,000 living in a small New England city. The population is composed of 7,700 Dominicans, 3,300 Puerto Ricans and 1,000 Guatemalans. The origins of the rest are scattered throughout Latin America. The focus will be on representatives of the three major groupings. They are members of the working class and migrated to the United States in the 1960s and 1970s in search of a better future. They live in the south and west sides of the city which they share with a largely black population. Health services in the neighborhood include two general hospitals, two community health centers, and for alcoholism a detoxification unit and a long-term residential setting (a halfway house) where people live and receive treatment often while also holding jobs.

CULTURAL FORMS OF TREATMENT

For those whose drinking has reached serious proportions either to the drinker or those who know him, there are varied forms of treatment for alcoholism in the Hispanic community that have nothing to do with health services. While they differ for Dominicans, Guatemalans, and Puerto Ricans, they are basically similar in that each group contextualizes alcoholism problems as part of a larger social or spiritual problem. Some of the alternative approaches are summarized below by presenting a typical case for each national group.

Overall, attitudes toward drinking in the Hispanic community discourage immoderate use and, therefore, serve preventive functions. There is no mutual agreement upon definition or impression of an alcoholic, but heavy drinking is sure to earn the disapproval of neighbors, family, and friends. Such behavior is associated with self-indulgent expenditures that deplete funds more properly applied to maintaining one's family. The alternatives used to describe habitual drinkers include not being *serio* (serious), being given to *adventurar,* and being *picaros* (unruly people) and *sin verguenzas* (those without shame).

As well, Hispanos express opinions about the special dangers of drinking for their people. Hispanos, they say, get out of control when drinking, far more so than for *la raza blanca* (white people). Casual mention of certain bars which are known to be Hispanic bars provoke stories of the dangers in these places. These stories include accounts of fights, shootings, and deaths on account of someone going berserk.

A Dominican Case

Paco (age fifty-two) had been a hard drinker in the Dominican Republic, and his pattern of drinking continued when he migrated to New York City in the mid-1960s, despite the problems it caused him there: fights on the street, discord with his wife that ultimately led to their separation, drinking so frequent that it dissipated most of his earnings. The notion that heavy drinking was socially unacceptable had not entered his mind; heavy drinking was the norm in the Dominican Republic, and not viewed as deviant behavior. However, on arriving in "Newtown" (a fictitious name, but a real town) and, once again, being reunited with his brothers, Paco found the rules of his culture changing. Instead of spending their money on immediate gratifications, Dominicans in Newtown were saving and conserving, sending money back home, buying houses, drinking less, and generally adopting a more austere mode of life. Significant for Paco was the attitude of his brothers who, in this new social and economic climate, refused to closely associate with him and openly criticized his indulgence in alcohol. Because of increasing isolation from his family, Paco began to reconsider his mode of life and to reevaluate his own position in a migrant Dominican culture becoming increasingly ascetic. His brothers promoted his attendance at a Catholic church, with its charismatic movement. This eventually supplied him with a moral orientation that relegated drinking to a vice and underscored the importance of a Christian life as one free of vice.

A Puerto Rican Case

Pedro started drinking at the age of thirteen at a small countryside bar owned by his stepfather. As a maturing adult, he began to drink regularly and heavily after work with other laboring men—a pattern more American than Hispanic—continuing to his current age of thirty-eight. While frequenting bars in Newtown, he came into increasing contact with Americans, some of whom began supplying him with mood-modifying drugs—euphoriants and barbiturates. One night after drinking, he felt stomach distress and a profound nervousness; he went to a hospital emergency room where his obvious anxiety prompted the attending physician to refer him to the hospital's psychiatric department for an appointment. Pedro returned to keep his appointment. He talked things over with the psychiatrist; they discussed "family problems" (a term Pedro used to locate the cause of his distress), and the psychiatrist prescribed librium and told Pedro to return in a week. He returned and reported that his distress had abated with the help of the pills. It was decided that there was no need for Pedro to return. Pedro's drinking appeared not to precipitate any further search for assistance until several months later when, in a bar, he heard a calling from Jesus and a welling up inside of feelings of faith and the need for prayer. He went to one of the local Pentecostal churches where he "accepted Christ" and pledged himself to a life with God. I met Pedro some four months after his religious awakening, and he reported that he had been sober consistently during this time and that he was regularly attending church. Pedro remained affiliated with the church, and for a year he was abstinent. Following this, he began drinking again in a manner that he describes as far more moderate.

A Guatemalan Case

Leon, in his late thirties, arrived from Guatemala after his life had fallen into disarray as a result of alcoholism. He had a series of job failures that constituted such a poor record of work performance that he found it impossible to find work paying a decent wage. Additionally, his drinking led to unresolvable ruptures in his family relationships. Having few options left, he journeyed north without family or friends and came to Newtown where he knew people. He eventually gravitated to Alcoholics Anonymous (AA).

His membership in AA in Newtown was not his first experience with this institution. He had been an AA member in Guatemala for a year but had lapsed back into drinking. At a party in Newtown, Leon was drinking heavily and, by his own account, was acting very unruly. Another Guatemalan approached him, said that Leon had a problem with his drinking and suggested that he join AA. The idea was again proposed to Leon several days later by this same person, who then made it his business to recruit Leon into his AA group. That man became his AA "sponsor," encouraging his sobriety and sustaining his commitment to AA. Leon has been in AA for the past year and a half.

Discussion of the Cases

While careers in treatment and recuperation can be very different, a common denominator among these cases is found in the care that is mediated by one's network of social relations and in the fact that behavior change salutory to health is so influenced. Among Dominicans, family members remain in close contact; they are concerned about deviant behavior and exert moral suasion. The change in norms of the Dominican community has inspired close scrutiny of behavior. The Catholic church echoes the changing cultural outlook and provides an orientation for personal change.

Puerto Ricans, by contrast, have far less involvement by extended family in their personal crises and rely far more on government-administered institutions for personal support and guidance. Alternatively, being wrenched out of a life of drinking by a calling to the Pentecostal church is relatively common in this city where five Pentecostal churches, each almost exclusively populated by Puerto Ricans, bring about an emotionally charged redefinition of one's life amidst others who likewise pledge themselves to a swift and radical break with drinking, dancing, and smoking—behaviors considered vices by the Pentecostals. Here they choose to entrench themselves in a closely knit and allegedly healing community of the church.

Guatemalans are another distinctive community by virtue of there being a preponderance of males who migrate to the United States and to Newtown without family. Companionship as well as psychological and economic assistance are supplied, when needed, by strong friendships which bind Guatemalans together in a network of predominantly male relationships. Among a group that is almost exclusively Guatemalan, it is not surprising that AA reached out to Leon. Guatemalan AA members make it their business to help fellow Guatemalans. Neither is it surprising that the idiom of assistance is AA as opposed to the church or psychiatric treatment. The presence of AA in Guatemala is considerable; tens of thousands have become at least nominal members after their political leadership affirmed the value of AA in the early 1960s.

COMMUNITY-BASED CARE

The development of community-based health care centers was a major initiative in health care reform developed as part of Lyndon Johnson's Great Society Program. It aimed to reach twenty-five million people who were without access to health care because of geographic or economic obstacles. Community-based centers were set up to be congenial and receptive to communities and their cultures. In certain respects this has been borne out, and the response of Hispanic communities in the country has shown considerable increase in volume of usage. Yet the content and quality of this usage has been undermined by the overwhelming influence of medical culture.

It was found that in the absence of neighborhood facilities, the volume of usage by Hispanos is far less than that of non-Hispanos. With the innovation of community centers and the removal of financial barriers, the rate of usage was equal to or greater than that of Anglos (Lee n.d.; Harwood 1981:452; Roberts and Lee 1980).

Analyses of utilization reveal that the emphasis on curative versus preventive health care does not change. There is merely more curative medicine reaching people. In Newtown, 90 percent of all Hispanic visits are for sick children or obstetric visits close to full term. There is a very low rate of well-child and early pregnancy visits in Newtown, and this is part of a nationwide pattern (Gaveria, Stern, and Schensul 1982; Guerra 1980; Harwood 1981:452–53; Hoppe and Heller 1975).

There is clearly a broad potential for preventive activities in many types of care, as would be helpful with people who have drinking problems. The potential exists because of the Hispanic residents who work in the center. They know the Hispanic community and are known by it. They are receptive to local customs and to the patients' expectations. They gain the confidence of the community's members. However, cultural expectations and norms of the community centers weaken an alliance between a center and its neighborhood. Consequently, the impetus to visit the center is mostly when the need is so strongly felt that people overlook their emotional discomfort with the setting.

Cultural differences between the clinic and the patient body discourage the casual consultation that would bear on matters of life-style. Pertinent cultural features describing Hispanos and Newtown clinics include (1) the bureaucratic routines, (2) the absence of *personalismo* (or personalism) in the clinic-patient relations, and (3) the patient expectations of a more rudimentary medicine, or *medicina empirica*.

1. Bureaucratic routines: Bureaucratic routines of the community health centers strain any confidence that might otherwise develop with Hispanic patients. Relations between practitioners and patients in the country of the patient's origin are not nearly so full of paperwork. When patients are presented with long forms for medical histories and for reimbursement to the health care center, they become mistrustful and withhold information. A key administrator remarked: "Some are very caught up in misinformation. They don't tell us that they have Blue Cross coverage. . . . They don't even tell us they have a job. They want us to be their physician, but they don't want to tell us anything about their lives."

2. *Personalismo:* A most important facet in the traditional physician-provider relations was the creation of a personal relationship with the patient. Traditionally, physicians communicate concern and firsthand knowledge of the patient's life. At first, the neighborhood health centers had the social service staff who were able to give personal attentions to patients. When needed, they made home visits, transported patients to the hospital, even accompanied them on visits to the welfare office. Patients responded to these attentions quite favorably, no doubt associating them with noninstitutional, informal care giving that is usually provided by family and friends.

When, in the mid-1970s, the government drastically reduced the budget for community health centers, patients became disaffected with the centers, finding there an impersonal quality, not dissimilar from the many other institutions Hispanos have come to know in the United States.

3. *Medicina empirica:* The Hispanic population generally had little confidence in the quality of care. The attitude was a continuation of attitudes toward medicine that they had developed in their country of origin.

In the Dominican Republic, the primary care offered in rural areas is wryly described as *medicina empirica,* or empirical medicine. In practice, this means that physicians prescribe medicines without a completely clear idea of the disorder. Diagnoses are confirmed or rejected based on the patient's response to medication. In the absence of funds and facilities for diagnostic tests, this is the only practicable form of treatment. Should a medication not prove effective, then another is tried with the presumption that the problem was other than expected.

The patient, however, is quick to try another doctor if the problem does not readily disappear. Or, the patient might turn to an herbalist if it was felt the doctor's medicine could not bring results. Patients expect results, and quickly. The unwillingness to stick with one doctor, for even a short time, confounds Dominican doctors. They speak of the *idiosincrasia* of the Dominican peasant. No less surprised were the staffs of the health centers. One administrator remarked that their tendency is to follow many physicians. Mothers make frequent and unwarranted use of the emergency room, "then they come here." Later they will change their pattern of use. "Now there is a migration of the Hispanic population from the center across town to us."

What in Newtown appears to be a fickle or irrational attitude and sometimes an abuse of the health care system is a very rational strategy for dealing with illness and a medical system without the laboratory technology found in the United States. However, the health care staff can only perceive the anxieties and lack of confidence which they can neither allay nor understand.

When Alcohol is Discussed

Hispanic patients relate well with the Hispanic nurses, nurses' aides, and clerical staff. Most health problems come first to their attention. Alcoholism is not an exception. Patients freely reveal that an injury was the result of the drunken rage of a brother or husband but they would not dare tell the same to a non-Hispanic worker.

The trust in the Hispanic health care worker applies equally as well outside the health care center. The richest flow of information about alcohol problems is transmitted in the home and on the street. Merely being an acquaintance of the health center staff is sufficient basis to talk over problems. Despite the potential usefulness and willingness of the Hispanic worker to help others with alcohol problems, the clinic's set-up makes it very difficult. When staff learn about a problem with drinking, they recommend a return visit to talk with the physician who is an expert on alcohol problems. When the matter is deferred to the moment when the physician or specialist is on hand, the concerned relative or friend of the alcoholic, or the alcoholic himself, will simply not show up. The Hispanic health care worker has no training, and no authority, to offer advice and is reluctant to do so. Consequently, there is no help forthcoming when it is sought.

HOSPITAL CARE

The trend in hospitals has been to subsume community-based care in their ambulatory clinics and to merge with smaller community hospitals. The trend toward more complex and bureaucratic structures in hospital care has triumphed because decision makers in these structures have adopted reform measures for their own ends that would have alternatively been used to expand community-based centers. The hospital model has digested reforms meant for community-level care and has used them to sustain themselves. A case in point is the development of specialty hospitals, specifically for alcoholics when the general hospital could not accommodate their treatment.

Before the Reform

Before the reform of care there was no time or interest in prevention or treatment of alcoholism. Alcoholism was simply not a medical problem. In Newtown, the emergency rooms of the two general hospitals did treat victims of accidents or fights that occurred while drinking. The nurses and physicians do recognize the obvious relation between drunkenness and trauma, but the cause of trauma is not investigated. A patient's drinking problems are just not seen as significant, for Hispanos as well as non-Hispanos. One nurse reported to me, "Like everyone else, [Hispanos] come in after a fight with liquor on their breath; however, the single problem is never especially alcohol." And they will treat the presenting problem, not the underlying one.

Nevertheless, inpatient nurses see alcohol problems all the time. A supervisor reports: "I bet you dollars to donuts that any nurse can go down the hall and identify each person who has an alcohol problem.

But they figure that's not what he's here for and that he's got enough problems. . . . The patient is here for one problem, he doesn't need another."

Hospital personnel viewed drinking problems as the proper concern of social workers, along with other problems that suggest noncompliant or "bad" patients. Nurses will call a social worker when a patient is particularly disruptive. Predictably, social workers feel slighted. One summed up the situation: "We get all the dumps. We're the garbage pail. A person can be an amputee and if he's crawling off in the corner of the room, the nurses will say there's no problem. We're not needed then; but if he's yelling and screaming, then they call us. We have to manage what they can't handle."

The First Reforms

The major reform in the treatment of alcoholism was the legislation to create the National Institute of Alcohol Abuse and Alcoholism.[2] The law plainly described alcoholism as "an illness requiring treatment and rehabilitation . . . through the assistance of a broad range of community health and social service agencies." The legislation made provision for the funding of state-level programs if state-level government enacted similar legislation seeking to handle alcohol abuse and alcoholism through treatment and prevention and not through the criminal justice system.

Newtown was affected by the state's having passed a "public inebriate" law protecting the public drunk from criminal prosecution. And the state opened an inpatient center where people could simply sober up and leave the next day or, alternatively, detoxify for about five days. This program was set up to treat "public inebriates and skid row inhabitants," according to its director. The state also opened a halfway house.

Hispanos and the First Reforms

Although federal and state laws unquestionably provided the foundation for the development of institutions to care for the poor, and federal legislation did result in some treatment to the poor, nonetheless the Hispanic community was largely unaffected.

There were, however, five Hispanos—all Puerto Rican—who previously would have come under the jurisdiction of the criminal justice system. With the reforms, they were placed under the newly developed services of the sobering up and detoxification units and the halfway house. These five had fallen into the "revolving door pattern" of drunken sprees, sometimes being picked up by the police and taken to treatment or arriving there voluntarily, and quite often residing in the halfway house in this or another state for stretches of several months. Partially, the stated objectives of the law were achieved; these five were no longer subject to the criminal justice system. But instead, they became the state's dependants. They were good patients, participating in all the treatment; they were supplied with food, housing, and welfare. The services reached only those whose problems were most extreme, difficult to resolve, and clearly vexing to the criminal justice system. Insofar as the Hispanic community was concerned, the reforms simply converted a criminal justice problem into a health care problem.

The Beneficiaries of Reform

The reforms of the treatment of alcoholism resulted in an increased involvement by health services. This meant that the treatment itself was fashioned on the medical paradigm, one curative, specialized, clinic-based, and isolated from social conditions.

The paradigm and the subsuming of alcoholism under a disease classification meant that various interests in the health care system would respond to the opportunities to offer treatment. The development of a treatment industry for alcoholism is only in some small way the result of structurally dominant sectors pursuing their own interests. The basic nature of our understanding of a medical problem means that the full complement of capital and labor resources will be brought to bear on the problem. The degree to which certain sectors of society are excluded is indeed a political-economic phenomenon. The emphasis and style of treatment, however, is intrinsic to the health care/medical paradigm and the pattern is being reproduced in socialist economies as well as capitalist ones.

In the past fourteen years following the passage of federal legislation, inpatient treatment centers have been established voluntarily by corporations and by government institutions. Today, there are about twenty-five hundred such centers. Treatment centers, private and public, became actively involved in public education, making extensive efforts to educate the public about alcoholism being a treatable disease. Eventually public education about alcoholism became subsumed under the marketing plans of treatment institutions in order to attract new patients. Finally, those viewing and promoting the idea of alcoholism as a treatable disease sought legislation to assure that third-party health insurers such as Blue Cross/Blue Shield would pay for treatment of alcoholism like they pay for treatment of other diseases.

In Newtown and in other communities in the state, efforts were made to pass laws requiring financial reimbursement for alcoholism treatment. Physicians and health care professionals with a commitment to treat alcoholics joined lay people with a concern for alcoholism in successfully mounting letter-writing campaigns, informal lobbying, and public testimony that convinced the state legislature to require employers to purchase health plans that included payment for rehabilitation for alcoholism.

Shortly before the law was passed, an alcoholism rehabilitation center was opened, and two opened afterwards. The cost of treatment is $150 to $250 per day in programs that last from thirty to thirty-four days. Those who are not covered by health insurance plans and are unable to pay for themselves may receive their alcoholism treatment in the detoxification center and the halfway house. Some limited number may enter treatment in one of the three new rehabilitation centers. The state set aside $400,000 for treatment in the three private institutions—quite a small sum since, in effect, it is just 1 percent of the total potential revenues of the combined centers. Clearly, this sum cannot cover potential demand nor a representative sample of the population. In the four years in which the centers have operated, only two Hispanos from Newtown have been admitted.

Throughout the country, the combined developments of the legitization of alcoholism as a disease and treatable condition, of the passage of laws decriminalizing drunkenness and providing for related health care, and of the development of alcoholism centers are all dramatic outcomes of a reform in health care which have had little impact on the conduct of general hospital care or on community health. In short, the reform simply grafted a rather specialized form of hospital care onto the existing setup of hospital care.

Despite the spectacular growth of inpatient care, choice of treatment is not based on evidence of positive clinical outcome. Nor is it a choice based on assessment of benefits relative to scarce capital resources to pay for care. One scholarly review of studies of inpatient versus outpatient treatment finds no advantage accruing from inpatient versus outpatient care. However, inpatient care is far more expensive. Despite this, the reviewer remarked that inpatient care "remains the cornerstone of service delivery in the alcoholism field" (Annis 1985–86:109).

A review of the costs and benefits of alcoholism treatment was undertaken by the Office of Technology Assessment (1983). Here, too, no sound justification was found for the trend to increased patient care even though the "trend is to increased coverage of free standing centers [and] provision of treatment equal to that for other diseases" (OTA 1983:73). The more affluent sectors of society, those with third-party insurance, are increasingly the greater share of consumers of services. The percentage of the total treatment costs borne by private third-party health insurers was 56.2 percent in 1979 and rose to 65 percent in 1982 (NIAAA 1983). Ownership of the alcoholism treatment is increasing in the hands of private for-profit corporations, increasing 48 percent between 1978 and 1982. The private not-for-profit alcoholism centers stayed about the same with a 1.2 percent increase, and the government-owned centers decreased 9.9 percent (NIAAA 1983). The data are taken from surveys completed every three years. The most recent survey, as yet unpublished, reveals a close to three-fold increase in the number of private for-profit alcoholism treatment centers.

DISCUSSION

The trend of alcoholism treatment reflects health care in general, some among its features being to rely on curative and not preventive care, to rely on higher cost modes of treatment, and to favor those who can pay more. The shift in paradigm from a criminal to a medical problem meant that medical institutions and norms would structure clinical strategies as well as patient demand for the services. The cultural paradigm, on the other hand, structures public censure, moral suasion, and spirituality that will address alcoholism. The cultural paradigm understands alcoholism as a social, moral, and spiritual problem. The medical paradigm is likely to find spiritual and moral difficulties being the logical outcome of alcoholism. The first is centered on an existential condition; the second on a purported disease.

When Dominicans encourage church attendance for someone who might be viewed as having a drinking problem, the objective is to change a way of life that is considered irresponsible, out of phase with progress, and, more importantly, without strength of purpose provided by believing in Jesus. Protestant Pentecostals promote deliverance from a variety of spiritual transgressions such as alcohol, drugs, smoking, dancing, and welfare. Treatment in this case is a total change of life; the absence of alcohol is just one part. When Guatemalans construe their problems as specifically related to alcohol, it is contextualized within symbols and ideas specific to and satisfying within their culture.

Indigenous forms of treatment are not the panacea. They attract only a small portion of the community who might benefit. One's personality, social network, and religious conviction will all influence both whether or not he uses the local resources, and his perceived need for help. Strategies for prevention and early treatment may be culled from several sources. The experience in community health centers suggests that social affiliation, based on mutual cultural understandings, is most effective in bringing drinking problems to light. Indigenous treatment indicates that one's behavior can be influenced in a culturally syntonic fashion while influencing those aspects of life-style impinging on health. In contradistinction, the presence of the health care system with its inclination to distinguish between the person and his problem, to isolate care from daily life, and to focus on cure undermines the therapeutic alliance that can be created within a community or cultural context.

It would be inaccurate to say that medical and health care overlook cultural differences. The problems in delivering alcoholism treatment to Hispanos are indeed recognized, but they are assessed from a commitment to the health care paradigm. Instead of finding health services remiss in treating Hispanic drinking problems, social scientists writing from the medical viewpoint find Hispanos laden with machismo preventing them from admitting weakness and accepting needed help; to make matters worse, this machismo also underlies the urge for drinking bouts.[3] Curiously, if an Anglo resists treatment or is prone to binge drinking, the difficulties are ascribed to the nature of the disease of alcoholism.

Bringing care for alcoholism to Hispanos will not be easily achieved through health care reforms. At best, bureaucratic reforms simply increase access to a system of curative care that is most successful when the patient body is culturally similar to the health care providers. Even if true reform did take place and socioeconomic inequalities were removed as Alford implies they need be, we would still be left with a curative and medical approach to a problem that is, in its roots and branches, behavioral. The undercurrent of thinking in medicine and in Alford's critique is that problems contextualized under health care systems approached from the medical paradigm should stay within the health care system paradigm; simply, care ought to be more equitably distributed. Alternatively, I suggest that prevention and many nonmedical treatment strategies could be contextualized broadly within the life of a people in their recreational, political, economic, and religious institutions. The strategies might include education, avoidance of alcohol for the alcoholic, monitoring diet and nutrition for those with cardiovascular problems, exercise, and smoking cessation programs.

Those responsible for health care policy are generally agreed that health care financing for many chronic diseases is placing increasingly heavy burdens on our economy. Continually, questions are posed as to how to contain costs. I can think of no better resolution than to interpolate much of care, particularly preventive, in community-based institutions so as to respond to the community's expectations and expressed needs. This will undoubtedly be most valuable in cases of traditional urban-ethnic groups.

The problems associated with alcoholism treatment, and with urban Hispanos, reflect the larger realities and difficulties of health care reform. Our traditional ethnic groups give us examples of populations that are less dressed up for compliance with the routines of health care. Traditional ethnic groups and their indigenous systems suggest most graphically how caring for health need not be dependent on reforms and on unresponsive bureaucratic institutions. Instead, their indigenous forms of treatment suggest fruitful alternatives and ways of thinking about how we may best care for ourselves.

NOTES

1. Much of the data for this paper was collected while a fellow in the NIAAA Program in Social Science Research Training on Alcohol, Grant No. T32 AA 0713105 sponsored by the Department of Anthropology, Brown University. Data from the Dominican Republic are culled from work as a Fulbright fellow there in 1980 and as Research Associate of the Museo del Hombre Dominicano in June through August 1983.

2. The Comprehensive Alcohol Abuse and Alcoholism Prevention Treatment and Rehabilitation Act of 1970.

3. Abad and Suarez 1975; Caste 1979, Caste and Blodgett 1981; Galbis 1977; Lopez Blanco 1980; Meadow and Stoker 1965; Panitz et al. 1983; Rodríguez and Rodríguez 1977; Simpson and Simpson 1978–79; Trevino 1979.

Failing Health and New Prescriptions: Community-Based Approaches to Environmental Risks

Richard A. Couto

We are increasingly familiar with a litany of chemicals and sub-stances that make our workplaces, schools, homes, food, water, and air suspect because of their possible adverse effect on our health. These chemicals and substances, some with initials to circumvent their com-plex names, make clear that health and illness are rooted in the every-day lives of people. The threat of these chemicals and substances intro-duces us to areas of failing health where scientific knowledge has clear limits and where questions of health and illness are obviously political and economic matters. These concerns relate to and substantiate recent criticisms of the American health care system and invite more radical analysis relating health care and illness directly to other economic and political issues.

Robert Alford's analysis of the American health care system offers us a means to identify the boundaries of health and health care analysis and how and why environmental health risks expand them. Before the issue of environmental toxicants gained national attention, Alford identified the structural interests of health professionals and planners as dominant and the structural interests of the general population as re-pressed in decisions and conflicts related to the allocation of health care resources. He offered occupational health as an instance of an underdeveloped health issue because of the repressed interests of workers (Alford 1975:16). The instances of conflict over environmen-tal health risks, which we will review, have characteristics similar to the conflicts between repressed and dominant structural interests over the allocation of health care resources.

Alford's analytical framework fits conflicts over occupational and environmental health issues well, though not precisely. One essential distinguishing characteristic of conflicts over environmental health is that they are conflicts over the allocation of health risks and not health resources. I shall draw on a controversy over an environmental health risk to exemplify a conflict between repressed and dominant structural interests and suggest a pattern of events in environmental health risk conflicts. I will emphasize one element of that pattern, a community-conducted health risk assessment. Finally, I will suggest that environmental health issues require that we extend Alford's analysis of health issues and perhaps extend our definition of health as well.

THE PATTERN OF CONFLICT OVER ENVIRONMENTAL HEALTH RISKS

Yellow Creek is in rural Bell County, which is near the southeast corner of Kentucky on the Tennessee and Virginia borders. The creek begins at a clean water source, Fern Lake, which provides Middlesboro, the county seat, its water. It empties into the Cumberland River as a polluted stream. Much of the pollution in Yellow Creek comes from Middlesboro's sewage treatment plant, which receives both residential and industrial wastes. The Middlesboro Tanning Company is the main contributor of industrial wastewater. It discharges approximately 750,000 gallons per day to the sewage treatment plant. In 1965, the tannery began using the blue chrome tanning process which requires the use of over 250 chemicals and metals. Prior to that, the process involved vegetable dyes which were biodegradable. The sewage treatment plant is a conventional secondary treatment facility and is incapable of properly treating the tannery's wastewater. Moreover, the toxic and corrosive nature of the tannery waste has damaged the plant to the point that it sometimes cannot even treat the residential wastes adequately. Therefore, untreated or poorly treated residential and industrial waste has been discharged into Yellow Creek. The Kentucky Bureau of Environmental Protection and the United States Environmental Protection Agency (EPA) concluded that the pollution had significantly harmed aquatic life along the creek (Kentucky Bureau of Environmental Protection 1980; U.S. Environmental Protection Agency 1981). In addition, a study by a private agency documented contamination of the creek sediment with cadmium, chromium, and lead (Polansky 1981).

Events along Yellow Creek replicate the events that have occurred elsewhere and suggest events to come in many other places. The pattern includes three sets of actors. The first is that of the community at risk, for example, the people who live along Yellow Creek. The second and third sets are part of the community of calculation. One part of this group is the community of consequence calculation—officials, both public and private, who allocate resources related to environmental health risks including the pollutants and toxicants themselves. The other actor is the community of probability calculation, i.e., epidemiologists. The important distinction among the groups is their structural interest, the primary economic and political foundations of their positions, which conflicts over environmental health often expose.

Yellow Creek residents and people in similar situations begin with shared evidence of obvious pollution. At Yellow Creek, people have witnessed fish kills in the creek for years. The fish would pack together so tightly to escape the "tan ooze" which depletes the oxygen in the creek's water that they would actually dam up the water of the creek. Love Canal residents experienced black sludge oozing out of cinder block walls and in one case a fiberglass pool was pushed up two feet out of its hole in the ground. There are more subtle measures which local people take as evidence of pollution. These include the disappearance of small animals such as rabbits and woodchucks from the area and the corrosion of screens and other metal or wood in places where people work or live. Other measures include trees and shrubs turning brown and shedding leaves early and in some cases losing leaves on one side but not the other. This street-wise or creek-side environmental monitoring proceeds independently of an individual awareness of serious and unusual health problems. For example, some couples try to have children without success. Other couples experience miscarriages, stillbirths, or infants with birth defects. Cancer afflicts old and young people. Still other people may complain of problems with specific organs, frequent dizziness, or difficulty with breathing. One Yellow Creek resident permitted his livestock to drink from the creek after his well ran dry only to see thirty-three pigs, four goats, and seven cows die shortly thereafter.

Sooner or later someone offers an intuitive judgment that there are health problems which are common, that the incidence of these problems is higher than expected, and that the problems are related to some common source, which is generally suspected to be the pollution, if it is known. This initial common sense epidemiology is most often the outgrowth of neighborliness or worker comradery such as conversations of people as they share a ride somewhere or a break from work. For example, in Yellow Creek a conversation among teenagers about the common concern of their parents brought their parents together. In Woburn, Massachusetts, a mother whose son had been diagnosed as having leukemia knew of two other children near her with leukemia and shared her suspicion that this was an abnormally high incidence with an Episcopalian priest who had provided her transportation to the hospital (Young 1983:19).

Based on this judgment, a few people organize and begin to take action. They conduct research on what has happened—often this is the collection of anecdotes of the pollution problem, health problems of residents, previous efforts people made to do something about the pollution, and pertinent medical advice and information people have received. This initial effort convinces the residents that they are dealing with a potentially serious problem which is common to many of their neighbors.

Shortly after organizing, people seek local help. A delegation is sent to a mayor, a county judge, or a board of health. This is when the community at risk first meets the community which calculates the consequence of dealing with the risk. There is a wide degree of reaction. In Trianna, Alabama, the mayor led the town's citizens in doing something about their DDT poisoning from the water and fish of Indian Creek (Reynolds 1980). Far more often, however, the community at risk encounters opposition rather than assistance from those who calculate consequence. There is first of all a denial of the problem, then a denial that the problem is serious, and then some attribution of the problem to the life-style and habits of the people who are at risk. Specifically, explanations were made at Yellow Creek that the livestock could have died from sunstroke and heart attacks; residents who asked for some action on pollution or toxicants were said to have grudges against the tannery related to past employment; and residents' concern for health was belittled if they smoked or were overweight.

These reactions are the expressions of a concern with the consequence of taking action regarding the source of pollution: the plant will close, hundreds or thousands of jobs will be lost, and local government will lose an important source of tax revenues. This environmental blackmail takes different specific forms (Kazis and Grossman 1982). At Yellow Creek the tannery vice-president put it concisely. "The people have to evaluate what's more important—a few carp or the livelihood of the community" (Staub 1983:45).

This is the first time but not the last time that the citizens will find opposition to their efforts. Other officials at other levels of government may also oppose them. Brown and Allen observed this process in other communities and reported, "It is at this point that the initial shock of the existence of toxics takes a back seat to the outrage people experience as their officials do nothing" (Brown and Brown 1983:8). But the outrage is deeper than a reaction to inaction. The outrage is a reaction to an assertion or inference that a regrettable but necessary cost of industry and business is environmental damage and a threat to the health of the community at risk. The inaction seems a decision that nothing should or can be done about the problem at hand. This extraordinary inference or assertion precedes and stimulates a radical reaction of the community at risk in defense of other values. As one Middlesboro resident explained: "When Yellow Creek Concerned Citizens (YCCC) first got started I thought they were gonna close the tannery down. I thought we can't have that—there's gotta be a compromise so the creek can get cleaned up and the tannery can still run. Then the more I read about it, the more I thought, 'If the tannery has to go to clear up Yellow Creek, than the tannery has to go' " (Staub 1983:50).

An example of this reactive outrage is evidenced in the response of a young member of YCCC to an answer she received from the secretary of the head of the Kentucky Department of Natural Resources and Environmental Protection.

> We have an unusual number of hysterectomies and miscarriages and stuff like that around the creek. I asked her if I got married if she could guarantee my kids would be healthy. She said no, she couldn't guarantee that, nobody could. Her recommendation to me would be not to get married. I got slightly heated. . . .

She made quite a few people angry. We mentioned that the food in our gardens was contaminated. She said, "Don't have gardens. Go to the store and buy it." People around here are not rich. That's why we have gardens, to save money. What state official has the right to get up and say, "Okay, you have problems. Don't get married. Don't have a garden." You don't quit your everyday life. (Staub 1983:47)

Citizen groups began to take direct and firm action to acquire response from local officials and others to their initial requests. Residents at Love Canal held two EPA representatives hostage for five hours (Clark et al. 1980:56). YCCC members also reacted to what they termed "a runaround." They went in numbers to the Middlesboro City Council meeting and asked if the city was going to enforce the law which prohibited existing practices of the sewage treatment plant. No answer was offered at the meeting, so YCCC members informed the council they were not leaving without an answer and thus began a two week sit-in at city hall. YCCC members eventually gained an unsatisfactory response from the Middlesboro mayor—he would not enforce the law at that time—and ended their sit-in. YCCC took other forms of direct action which YCCC members understood others might consider militant and disapprove of because they had stood in similar judgment over others on the same matters previously. YCCC members surprised themselves by conducting the "radical" actions they had previously disapproved. Larry Wilson, president of YCCC, recounted a political and personal change as a result of the conflict over Yellow Creek.

My whole philosophy on life has changed. Back in the sixties when all the demonstrations were going on, anybody who told me that one day I'd be carrying a sign in front of a government building probably would have had to fight right there. Now I'm doing it and encouraging others to do it. I've got a better understanding of our political system and it scares the hell out of me. We've got the best political system in the world, but it's got one-sided. Our government revolves around huge corporations. . . .

My personal values have changed. Best thing I can leave my kids and my grandkids is a better society. Before it was money. Money doesn't mean a thing to me now. Peace of mind, a happy society where people are doing for instead of to is what it's all about.

If this is radical, then we'd be better off if the whole world was radical. (Staub 1983:46)

In this environment of heightened political conflict, violence may occur. At Yellow Creek, the mayor reported being shot at in his office; the following night a YCCC member reported being shot at in his truck; and later two officers of the YCCC reported being shot at while driving. Bullet holes and shattered glass testified amply that shots had been fired in every instance.

A lack of official response and the increased political sophistication and publicity citizens acquire as a result of the conflict eventually leads citizen groups to enlist other allies in their conflict. They form networks with other citizen leaders and citizen groups concerned with similar problems. Lessons of one group are shared with another, advice is exchanged and in some instances new coalitions are formed. By this time the group has also acquired the assistance of professionals from outside the community who are desirous to assist and often have some experience in working with similar groups and/or related issues. These professionals may include physicians, chemists, social scientists, environmentalists, or lawyers. Through these networks and with this assistance the conflict becomes much broader. Regional and even national media may cover the story, and representatives from the community at risk may testify before committees of their state legislature or even Congress.

The community of consequence calculation eventually challenges the community at risk to provide proof of a danger to human health. Such proof is necessary, they argue, to warrant the cost of pollution cleanup or to justify the dire consequences that might be associated with curtailing operation of the plant or mill that is the source of the pollution. Consequently, citizens groups consider acquiring additional information as a tactic to gain action from local, state, and federal officials. It is at this time that the community at risk becomes acquainted with the second portion of the community of calculation. These are epidemiologists who attempt to demonstrate the strength of associations between illness and pollution. The first lesson that members of the community at risk acquire about epidemiologists is that they are a scientific community with canons, strictures, procedures, and paradigms. The second lesson they acquire is that for all their rigor, epidemiologists are in their earliest stages of determining causal links between pollution and illness. There may be no registries listing the incidences of illness with which the community residents are concerned. Previous studies, if relevant at all to the existing pollutants, are not well organized and provide contradictory evidence if any evidence at all about thresholds and exposure rates. It thus becomes clear that the scientific community learns from people already exposed and that the community at risk will probably give to the community of probability calculation more information than they will receive from them. A final lesson that the community at risk acquires is that epidemiological studies are beyond their ability to conduct. They require too many professionals who are unavailable to them and whose services cost more money than a community group can afford.

It is at this point that a citizens' group may undertake, as YCCC did, a health risk assessment to determine the level of health and illness in a particular community and its relationship to pollution. These assessments are not epidemiological studies in a strict sense, but they are more than a collection of anecdotes. They are time–consuming and may very well require the energy of the community leaders and community members that might otherwise have gone into direct political action. On the other hand, direct political action leads to increased demands from the community of consequence calculation that a group substantiate its claims of damage to warrant official action, that the group, in effect, "put up or shut up."

In addition, as a consequence of some of the preliminary findings or self-assessments, official assessments are also undertaken. Here again, however, citizens confront the inadequacies of epidemiology. In Trianna, Alabama, for example, the Centers for Disease Control found conclusive evidence of DDT poisoning and even abnormally high levels of PCBs in the residents of the town. Trianna has a population with the highest reported levels of DDT in humans (Reynolds 1980). No one is quite sure what illness conditions to expect or which might be associated with these high levels of DDT. In Love Canal, one family discovered that the air quality in their cellar, which had been an individual problem for so many years, was a very substantial environmental problem; the exposure to this air, according to federal standards, should be limited to 2.4 minutes (Brown 1979:38). In Yellow Creek, the Centers for Disease Control conducted a study of leukemia at the request of state officials and in reaction to YCCC allegations of higher than normal rates of leukemia along the creek. The CDC study found a rate of leukemia four times what would be expected. Given the small numbers involved—two cases—this rate was not statistically significant ($p<.07$). CDC did recommend, however, a new water source and minimum exposure of the population to the water of Yellow Creek (Centers for Disease Control 1982).

The residents of Yellow Creek worked successfully with county officials for a federal grant to install a new water system for residents along the creek. This is indicative of the small victories that citizens acquire in their battles. The first and foremost victory is the recognition that the pollution problem is real and that it may pose a threat to health. The YCCC members acquired this victory when the board of health permitted signs along Yellow Creek indicating the danger of swimming or eating fish from the waters. In Trianna, the community was assisted with federal support in the establishment of a community garden to develop other sources of food than the fish in the creek which were heavily contaminated with DDT. In addition, Trianna, again with federal support, acquired a primary health care clinic to improve the health care available to local citizens. In addition to these small victories, citizens also acquire larger local victories. Out-of-court settlements with companies responsible for the pollution are often for a tiny fraction of the originally requested funds but represent some reimbursement for losses incurred. Generally, these settlements are worded to avoid any admission of guilt or liability, past or future, on the part of the companies or pollution sources for damage to the health of individuals. The YCCC gained a particularly significant victory in November 1983, when a political reform group in Middlesboro, which YCCC supported, acquired a working majority on the Middlesboro City Council in the election held that month. In addition, the EPA has started enforcement procedures as YCCC urged, but more slowly than YCCC wanted and without consistent resolve.

The victories of local groups, both big and small, should not disguise a process of dealing with particular problems and avoiding the larger systemic questions of who controls the environment, for what purpose, and the consequence on the health of those who live within it. The maximum control of a common and public environment by private interest at least cost to them is a consistent principle that is fought for in each instance by the different members of the community of consequence calculation. These interests have the most similar vested stakes in the consequence of the question as it is generally applied and have far superior resources to devote to the conflict over the question than local citizens who oppose them. This reminds us of Alford's observation on the different resources available to equal health advocates on the one hand, the professional monopolies and corporate rationalizers on the other hand, and "the quiet and continuous allocation of benefits to dominant structural interests" (Alford 1975:16).

HEALTH RISK ASSESSMENTS AND THE POLITICS OF PROBABILITY

The health risk assessment of the YCCC demonstrated statistically significant associations between reported illness conditions and exposure to creek water. Specifically, residents who use water from private wells in areas along Yellow Creek that are more prone to flooding reported higher rates of kidney ailments and illness conditions of the lower gastrointestinal tract. Residents also reported a statistically significant increase in miscarriages after 1970, which is five years after the heavy metals process was introduced at the tannery (Sherman and Couto 1984).

The health risk assessment which the YCCC conducted is important for reasons other than its findings. Its place in the pattern of conflict suggests that a health risk assessment is a unique part of the process of community mobilization around environmental health risks. The processes which precede it and follow it offer grounds for understanding the dominance of structural interests in environmental health and the political nature of environmental health risks and conflicts over them. Finally, the health risk assessment has important links to participatory research methodologies and critiques of established science.

The community-conducted health risk assessment at Yellow Creek was developed, conducted, and analyzed over a 2½ year period. The Health Survey Committee of the YCCC worked along with a Ph.D. in community psychology, an M.D. in pharmacology, a public interest group, and students provided by the Student Environmental Health Project of the Center for Health Services at Vanderbilt University. The survey was a long process and entailed the volunteer efforts of local residents and voluntary resources from several universities. The questionnaire was a combination of survey research methodology and community concern. Members of the Health Survey Committee of YCCC conducted the interviews at almost three hundred households involving almost one thousand people. The process of developing and conducting the survey was educational and important for mobilizing local resources. It slowed down and even became burdensome after the excitement of interviewing was finished and the tedium of coding and analysis began. In this regard the survey resembles most survey research efforts, but it represents a particular problem for this type of community-conducted survey. That is, the continued efforts of deciphering, coding, and analyzing responses requires the continued assistance of almost free university resources which are scarce for this type of work. This increase in professional participation results in a serious decline in community participation during this stage of assessment.

Like any survey, this assessment could neither prove nor disprove a hypothesis. The methodological problems and analytical shortcomings of the survey guaranteed that its findings would not be accepted as "scientific." Without question, improvements can be made on efforts such as the Yellow Creek health risk assessment. In Woburn, Massachusetts, for example, one group has conducted a study with the cooperation of the Harvard School of Public Health (Young 1983; Lagakos, Wessen, and Zelen 1984). This is an extensive study with the authority of the Harvard School of Public Health and a model for epidemiology. It may be a powerful help in this particular community's effort but it is not necessarily a model for communities at risk. First, such a study cannot be replicated easily. Some estimates of the cost of this study ran as high as $750,000. It is difficult to get universities, foundations, and community volunteers to coalesce to this extent time after time. For one reason, faculty members at universities are ordinarily reluctant to use their time on community surveys which fall outside or contradict the dominant pattern of rewards and resources for their promotion and prestige. Another reason this Woburn study may not be a model is that even this thorough study will be challenged for its findings and will involve the community at risk in an academic dispute on the scientific merits of the study.

Consequently, while we improve on past experience in community health risk assessments such as at Yellow Creek, we also need to articulate their lessons and make them more effective. The first lesson is that some form of health risk assessment is necessary and inevitable at some stage of a conflict over serious pollution. The second lesson is that these assessments vary in their expense and accessibility for community residents. Third, if they are kept inexpensive and under community direction, they are unlikely to achieve the status of epidemiology but may increase community organization. YCCC canvassers had a 99.5 percent response rate, for example, among almost three hundred households.

If the solutions to pollution problems were inexpensive and expedient, community-conducted health risk assessments would probably be adequate as reasonable measures to indicate that some remedial action to pollution should be taken. However, most solutions are complicated and expensive procedures, and their costs often require that the benefit of pollution control or the removal of toxicants be demonstrated to exceed the costs of these measures. This is why the preservation of human health becomes a factor in cost-benefit analysis. Once it becomes a factor, then the risk to human health must be calculated. Because rigorous epidemiological studies are ordinarily beyond the means of community groups to initiate, community groups devise their own assessments of risk.

We should take note of the politics of epidemiology as well as the politics of community health surveys. Epidemiology shares with other sciences a preference for doubt rather than asserting a false claim. Of the two types of false claims epidemiology can make, it would rather falsely claim no association between variables when there is one than claim an association when it does not exist. It seeks evidence to establish a level of confidence with which to reject a null hypothesis that variables are not related rather than to assert clearly that they are. Consequently, epidemiology has a conservative bias in drawing conclusions. This bias serves science and society well in many instances by demanding rigorous proof for any assertion. However, this bias conflicts with the need of a community at risk, which is a need for an assessment and calculation of what might happen, what is happening now, as well as what has happened. An analysis of already reported cases of illness for the statistical significance of their rates or associations with other factors addresses only the last part of the needs of a community at risk, although it is an important part of the cumulative process of science.

In addition to epidemiology's concern with its paradigms and integrity, epidemiology shares with other sciences the potential for mistakes and manipulation in studies of the relation of pollution and illness. Examples of information on risk include instances when risk was miscalculated in the case of DES (Brackbill and Berendes 1978); recalculated to acquire more assuring figures on nuclear reactor safety (Welch 1980); ignored in the case of formaldehyde (Ashford, Ryan, and Caldart 1983); or repressed as in the mercury contamination at Oak Ridge (*Tennessean* [Nashville] 1983a; 1983b; 1983c).

Epidemiology and community-conducted health risk assessments share a concern for the calculation of risk, which is a combination of probability and consequence. It is important to understand that they are two approaches to the question, How do we know what is the right and reasonable action to take in the face of uncertainty? Put in these terms, events along Yellow Creek are part of an enduring and complex human dilemma that has absorbed philosophers and moralists for a longer time than it has preoccupied epidemiologists (Nagel 1939). The evidence that epidemiologists require to achieve scientific statements of probability exceeds the evidence required to state that probably something should be done to eliminate or minimize a threat to health.

The degree of risk to human health does not need to be at statistically significant levels to require political action. The degree of risk does have to be such that a reasonable person would avoid it. Consequently, the important political test is not the findings of epidemiologists on the probability of the nonrandomness of an incidence of illness but the likelihood that a reasonable person, including members of the community of calculation, would take up residence with the community at risk and drink from and bathe in water from the Yellow Creek area or buy a house along Love Canal.

In distinguishing epidemiology from a health risk assessment, it is important to remember that the threat to health is distinct from incidence of illness. One may make reasonable judgments about the incidence of illness, but these are far more controversial than judgments about threats to health. Large court suits are won by proof of illness, not evidence of threats to health. The burden of proof in both matters is on the community at risk in both the court of law and the court of public opinion. To deal with this burden, a community at risk is ordinarily better off establishing reasonable grounds that there is a threat to health than attempting a scientifically rigorous investigation of the incidence of illness. This is because the conflict is essentially political, and the community at risk has limited resources which are more effectively used in shaping public awareness. Ordinarily, courts will only award the community at risk limited victories based on a threat to health anyway.

Given the limited resources of a community at risk, members of that community are better off conducting assessments of the health risks—changes in the environment, indications of toxic pollution, and reported conditions of illness—and demanding that official agencies conduct the more rigorous epidemiological studies. Another reason for requiring official agencies rather than the community at risk to do the epidemiology of illness is that illness caused by pollution is the most expensive aspect of the liability of companies and the most heavily contested. The community of consequence calculation takes all means possible to avoid liability for illness related to environmental hazards. The Johns-Manville Company recently reorganized in light of a pending bankruptcy given the number of claims against it for illness related to asbestos products. This action is an example of the lengths to which companies will go to avoid liability related to the damage to health from environmental hazards (Kelly 1982). The community at risk needs formidable allies to win a contest over toxic pollutants as a cause of a specific illness. It can be done, but the first and surest step for the community at risk is to conduct a health risk assessment of the probable threat to health and to demand and to monitor the epidemiological studies of others.

SOCIAL SCIENCE AND THE EXTENDED ANALYSIS
OF HEALTH

By way of summary and conclusion it may be useful to outline the ways in which we might apply and extend Alford's analysis to incorporate new and emerging issues on environmental health risks. First of all, Alford's basic point that health care reform and policy is a conflict between dominant and repressed structural interests remains central to conflicts over environmental health risks. The analysis that I have presented simply underscores the validity of understanding health policy disputes as grounds to critique the premises and assumptions of American pluralism, which is the central theoretical aspect of Alford's work. That is to say, the assumption that all interests are equal in the competition for health policy outcomes is refuted by the recent experience of community groups working on environmental issues as well as the earlier experiences of the equal health advocates.

We may revise Alford's analysis to better fit issues of environmental health risks. The major actors in Alford's analysis are the professional monopolist, corporate rationalizers, and the equal health advocates. What we have called the community of probability calculation, or epidemiologists, fits well the role and definition which Alford provided for professional monopolists (Alford 1975:194–200). Alford cited Friedson to describe a consequence in American health care due to the professional monopoly which is equally applicable to the consequence for epidemiology. "[Organized medicine] asserts its control over medical work at the same time its practitioners are too few to perform the work. It refuses to allow members of other occupations to program such work except in a position of subordination from which they can gain little satisfaction. It insists on its jurisdiction over everything related to that vague word 'health' " (Alford 1975:198–99).

The other actors in the conflicts over health and pollution, unlike the professional monopolists, need substantial reinterpretation. The community at risk is not a set of equal health advocates nor professional advocates for better distribution of health resources and health care. They are people at risk for illness from exposure to pollutants and are often directly involved in addressing that need. They are similar to equal health advocates in that their structural interest is repressed in the sense that, as we have seen clearly, "no social institutions or political mechanisms in the society insure that these interests are served" (Alford 1975:15). In fact, so few institutional resources are available to community residents that they have to expend vast amounts of energy and financial resources. For this reason it is common that leaders of such groups sometimes confess that if they had known what they were getting into they might not have made the effort (Young 1983:22). Members of the community at risk are also similar to the equal health advocates in that their position on health includes the prevention of illness and not merely its treatment.

As we distinguish the members of the community at risk from the professionals who comprise Alford's equal health advocates, we must remember that there are epidemiologists and physicians sympathetic and supportive of groups such as YCCC. Their role is very significant. They can lend great credence to community efforts to assess a health risk. However, in that very process they can relegate community residents to a minor role in the assessment process and shift the process from overtly political grounds to seemingly apolitical, scientific grounds. By inadvertently relegating community residents to a minor role and shifting grounds of the controversy, health professionals and epidemiologists replicate more precisely the role of the equal health advocates in Alford's analysis. This is almost inevitable if community residents, workers, or other affected groups seek to conduct epidemiology. The politics of epidemiology is such that epidemiology is what epidemiologists do. This is the reason for the distinction I have made between a community-conducted health risk assessment and epidemiology. That is, it does not take an epidemiologist to do a health risk assessment; it is far less costly and it is free of the controversy about whether or not it crosses the threshold of epidemiology. There are certainly grounds to claim that health risk assessments are epidemiology, but that debate is best left to the epidemiologists among the equal health advocates to resolve with their colleagues rather than to place community residents in yet another controversy within a conflict over health and pollution.

Based on conflicts over environmental health risks, we need to expand Alford's description of equal health advocates to include some element of the citizens' movement which Harry Boyte has identified. Health as a concept also needs to be expanded to incorporate some sense of community which Boyte sees as a core around which diverse citizens' movements revolve. "The citizen movements represent, indeed, an alternative popular democratic thread of insurgency in modern society. . . . It grows mainly in . . . those 'organic' relations that modern life has not completely collectivized, rationalized and refashioned in the image of the market place. And it incubates an alternative world view, different from the conventional vision of either the left or right" (Boyte 1980:xiv).

The expression of new realizations by YCCC members during the conflict along Yellow Creek gives Boyte's generalization a specific and accurate referent. In general, the "radical" nature of the citizens' effort defies political categorization of either Left or Right and is much more related to an organic sense of the fit of human beings and their environment. This fit of humans and their environment, which is part of community, is also part of the definition of health which Rene Dubos offered to us. He suggested that the real measure of health and disease "is the ability of the individual to function in a manner acceptable to himself and to the group of which he is a part" (Boyte 1980:214). Health is "the condition best suited to reach goals that each individual formulates for himself" (1980:228). Similarly, much of the work done on primary health care innovation in Third World countries by equal health advocates emphasizes health as "an expression, or spin-off, of a quietly functioning informed community" (Newell 1975:192; Morley, Rohde, and Williams 1983; Connor and Mullan 1982).

The emerging field of participatory research (Hall 1975; Fals Borda 1979) seems to be grounds on which to combine an emphasis on community with the need to acquire knowledge. More specifically and related to our concerns, participatory research and community health risk assessment have much in common. Participatory research needs to be refined on the basis of the strengths and limitations of instances like Yellow Creek, and instances of participatory research can better inform subsequent community health risk assessments.

The role of corporate rationalizers in conflicts over environmental health needs further elaboration and definition. This is because we are not concerned about the distribution or rationalization of existing or possible health *resources* but with the distribution and rationalization of *threats* to health and the cost of action to deal with those threats. The sources of those threats to health represent another element of the corporate sector in the American economy. Consequently, the conflicts over environmental health require a much more radical analysis of the determinants of health and illness than Alford provides.

Alford's suggestion that a class or institutional analysis rejects the assumption that health care as a problem can be isolated is not just one mode of analysis but the obvious starting point for the analysis of environmental health issues which have economic roots and political implications. Vincente Navarro (1976) points out that a common weakness of analysis of health and medicine is that social scientists begin with precisely the wrong assumption—that health is a policy sector somehow autonomous from the rest of society. Both Navarro and

Doyal (1979) offer analysis of health, health care, and medicine in terms of the economic and political character of capitalist society. Chalmers (1982) makes a point of epidemiology's limits because its scientific principles exclude class as a factor of analysis. Even the response to environmental problems indicates further the class and racial correlates of health and medicine in capitalist society. Licensed toxic waste dumps in the Southeast in 1982 were located in proximity to low income communities with a majority black population (General Accounting Office 1983).

The issues and conflicts surrounding community environmental health are an open invitation for the application of further critiques of American pluralism. The rich literature on symbolic uses in politics, non–decision making, and power offers elaboration on Alford's distinction between dominant and repressed structural interests (Couto 1975; Crenson 1971; Gaventa 1983; Lukes 1974). This literature and our experience with environmental conflicts invite deeper analysis of issues in American health care and American political life which have not reached the level of decision making. This literature helps us better understand why threats to health sometimes are ignored and what are the determinants of the resolution of conflict over those threats which do come to light.

Finally, the emerging issues and continuing conflicts of environmental health are grounds for the imagination of social science as C. Wright Mills described it. It is hard to conceive of an area of study where the political task of social science which Mills assigned it could be clearer; namely, to translate personal troubles into public issues and public issues into the terms of their human meaning for a variety of individuals (Mills 1950:187).

Diet and Agricultural Development: The Dietary Correlates of Changes in Agricultural Policies in a Mexican Community

Kathleen M. DeWalt

Hulse (1982) has recently argued that the failure to pay careful attention to the nutritional impact of food production and processing technology on the poor in less developed countries results in the formulation and implementation of food policy with little or no evidence to predict its consequences for nutritional status. Hulse was addressing the area of food science and postharvest processing specifically, but the argument is even more applicable to production policies. As Valdes (1983) points out, agricultural policy is not synonymous with food policy. Even if such policies exist, national agricultural goals and food policy may not be designed to meet the needs of small farmers.

The introduction of new crops and production technologies to small farmers is not nutritionally neutral. Unfortunately, evidence suggests that it has frequently not been positive, at least in terms of the small farm family. Fleuret and Fleuret (1980), in a review of nutrition, consumption, and agricultural development, conclude that few programs to improve the productivity of small farmers have had a positive impact on the nutritional status of their families. Some may have even contributed to a decline in nutritional status.

Changing crop choice and techniques of cultivation can contribute to changes in food availability and nutritional status in several ways. Perhaps the most controversial question is the effect of replacing subsistence crops with cash crops under the assumption that increases in income will enable the producer to purchase displaced foods. This assumption has not been clearly supported. Increasing income may provide a *different* diet, but not necessarily a *better* diet (DeWalt 1983a).

The applications of some technologies to the production of subsistence crops can result in a decline in crop diversity and consequently in dietary diversity. The elimination of unplanted food producing crops such as the edible wild plants that grow in the disturbed soils between rows of cultivated crops may also affect dietary adequacy. The value of displaced minor crops and uncultivated plants is often overlooked because these plants do not provide the bulk of energy as other crops do, but may be a major source of micronutrients (Messer 1972, 1977; DeWalt 1983b).

Finally, technologies requiring reallocation of labor may have dramatic effects on the nutritional status of family members. Some have argued that the commercialization of agriculture results in a diversion of food resources from nonproductive members of the household (ie. children) to productive members of the household (Gross and Underwood 1971; Fleuret and Fleuret 1980).

Despite this series of questions concerning the nutritional impact of agricultural policies encouraging the introduction of alternative techniques of production and new cropping patterns in small farm families, careful study of the nutritional impacts of agricultural change has rarely been carried out. In this paper I will examine the dietary and nutritional correlates of several decades of attempted agricultural policy change in a farming community in central Mexico.

Agricultural policy in Mexico in the late 1960s and early part of the 1970s was based on a classic notion of modernization (Hewitt de Alcantara 1976; DeWalt 1985). Policy was focused at increasing production through the expansion of infrastructure, the employment of "green revolution" technology, and the promotion of cash-generating crops for international trade and import substitution. The initial beneficiaries of the agricultural modernization were primarily larger landholders. The result was a dramatic expansion of production, first of food crops and later of export crops. Development of the small holder—the *ejidatario*—was approached with similar models of development. National policy emphasized the replacement of subsistence crops with cash crops both for the generation of cash for rural households and for import substitution on a national level. Despite the beliefs of agricultural change agents concerning the conservative nature of small cultivators, the agricultural policy climate created had dramatic impacts on the agricultural strategies of *ejidatarios*.

This paper examines the results of shifting agricultural strategies on the diets of *ejido* families in a community in the state of Mexico. A series of development projects undertaken in the region and the effects of these on the agricultural strategies of *ejido* households in a small community are outlined. The diets of a sample of community households are analyzed to see the effects of alternative agricultural strategies on diet.

AGRICULTURAL CHANGE IN THE VALLEY OF TEMASCALCINGO

The Valley of Temascalcingo, located in the central highlands of Mexico, is an agricultural area of substantial potential. The seventeen thousand hectares of land in the valley are divided into sixteen *ejidos* and distributed among approximately three thousand *ejidatarios*. There are also a few large private landholdings and a number of small private holdings. The land on the valley floor has been irrigated since colonial times. Land on hillsides is rain-fed but potentially cultivatable.

The small size of individual landholdings and the periodic flooding of the Lerma River have been major constraints to the realization of the productive potential of the area. Because of this potential, however, the Valley of Temascalcingo has been the site of a parade of development projects since land redistribution in the early 1930s. Shortly after land redistribution, a number of loans were provided for the purchase of oxen, plows, and other agricultural equipment by the newly formed Banco Ejidal. Unfortunately, officials sent by the bank to collect loan repayments pocketed the money. *Ejidatarios* were later harassed and jailed for nonpayment of debt obligations they had actually fulfilled. These experiences set the tone for all subsequent encounters with extralocal aid.

Another program dating from the early days of the formation of the *ejido* was an attempt to establish a sheep-raising industry in the valley. A number of purebred sheep were introduced without regard for their ability to adapt to the local climate. Development agents claim that many of these sheep were quickly killed and sold or eaten. The *ejidatarios* maintain, however, that the sheep were not accustomed to the climate and soon died. Some *ejidatarios* still owe money on the loans made for the purchase of the sheep. This program may not have been a total failure, however, as before dying or otherwise disappearing, some rams crossbred with native ewes, improving the local stock somewhat.

About 1950, a program designed to improve wheat crops in the region was introduced. An improved variety of wheat seed was distributed, along with fertilizer. Rather than increased yields, the *ejidatarios* found that their harvest was smaller than usual. Although agricultural engineers could say that the particular variety of seed used was inappropriate for the area, the *ejidatarios* concluded that improved varieties and fertilizers were of no value.

The Brigada Agropequaria, a government-funded technical assistance group consisting of agricultural extension workers, was headquartered in the former Hacienda Solís in the valley center in the 1950s and early 1960s. The *brigada* sponsored a number of projects, including the planting of fruit trees and vegetable gardens and beekeeping. At about this same time, the age-old problem of flooding became more desperate as the levee and drainage system maintained by the haciendas during the colonial period began to break down from neglect. For several years in a row, flooding by the Lerma River destroyed most of the maize crop.

In the early 1960s, the cabinet-level Secretariat for Hydraulic Resources (SRH) began a flood-control and irrigation project in the valley. The decision to take this action was surely aided by the prominent position of a local landholder who owned a large tract of land on the valley floor and who was at that time the Secretary (minister) of Hydraulic Resources.

The project, called Plan Lerma, was conceived of as a massive development project that crosscut political boundaries and included technical development of the physical environment through flood control and irrigation as well as the promotion of socioeconomic development through improved agricultural practices and household management. It was patterned after the development projects being carried out in the Papoloapan and Balsas river basins (Barkin and King 1970). The project was partially funded through international sources and included a number of different agencies. The Temascalcingo region was one of three regions in which Plan Lerma operated. Dams built upriver from the Temascalcingo area as well as the dredging of a new riverbed through the valley and the reinforcement of the river banks significantly improved the flooding problem. Drainage ditches were dredged and reinforced, and the irrigation system was improved and expanded.

The other development accomplishments of Plan Lerma were relatively modest. A small housing renovation project took place in one community; some fruit trees were distributed; technical advice on fertilizers, herbicides, insecticides, animal diseases, and other agricultural techniques were provided; and some cooking and nutrition classes were held.

The most ambitious program drawn up by Plan Lerma personnel was a scheme to transform the valley into a dairying region through the introduction of forage crops, purebred dairy cattle, and modern methods of animal husbandry. By 1971, however, the agency had decided to concentrate its funds and personnel in a different region of Mexico and left the valley.

In 1970, a program called Plan Maiz was active in the valley. The program, supported by the government of the State of Mexico, sought to apply "green revolution" technology to the production of maize. The goal of Plan Maiz was to improve maize production in Temascalcingo to the extent that subsistence needs would be exceeded and maize could serve as a cash crop for small farmers. Plan Maiz hoped to encourage the use of hybrid seed, mechanical cultivation, pesticides, and chemical fertilizers. This was to be accomplished by organizing *ejidatarios* to cooperatively plow large sections of land using tractors and extending large amounts of credit for the purchase of seed, chemical fertilizers, pesticides, and tractor rentals. A team of agricultural agents was available for technical assistance.

Maize production was significantly improved by Plan Maize, but *ejidatarios* maintained that improved production was not sufficient to pay off all the debts they had incurred. In 1971 a number of *ejidos*, including the research community, refused to participate in Plan Maiz, and by the following year the project and its aggressive project leader were gone. Plan Maiz did demonstrate the benefits of fertilizer, and in 1973 there was enough local interest that a small amount of credit for the purchase of fertilizer was made available.

In 1973 SRH was the major agency involved in development activities in the Temascalcingo region. Some work on the riverbed and irrigation system was continuing, although the huge investments of millions of pesos in technological improvement had had little discernable return in improved production or improvement in the standard of living. However, SRH continued to carry out the plans developed by Plan Lerma and was instrumental in developing a mix of grasses and clovers that grew well in the region and would support dairy and beef cattle. SRH planned to organize *ejidos* into dairying cooperatives in which land would be cooperatively planted in forage, large modern barns constructed, and cattle imported from other regions of Mexico and possibly Canada. By late 1974 several *ejidos* were persuaded to organize and sow forage crops, and credit was extended to build barns. Forage produced during the waiting period before the cattle arrived had a ready market and sold well.

By 1977 three dairy cooperatives were in operation and the fourth was awaiting the completion of the barn and the arrival of cattle. Milk production in the operating dairies was below expectations and the price even lower. Cooperatives were unable to produce a profit and could not pay back the huge debt incurred. Ironically, milk produced by these cooperatives was sold at a low price to pasturization companies outside the valley, while the demand for raw milk within the valley was high and the local price significantly higher. None of the companies buying the milk marketed the pasturized product in Temascalcingo.

The fourth cooperative, located in the community under study here, was never operational. The barn was never completed and cattle never arrived. By 1982 all of the dairy cooperatives had been abandoned and the barns remained quiet and empty.

Several other agencies with somewhat different approaches to agricultural change and development have also worked in the area. The agency for the Integrated Development of the Family (DIF)—an arm of the Mexican Institute for Assistance to Children (IMAN), which operates an internationally known children's hospital in Mexico City—occupied the former Hacienda Solís from about 1977 to 1980. The original intent of DIF in Temascalcingo was to study the effects on the health of children of the transformation of a maize-producing area to a dairying region.

When it became clear that the expected transformation was not to occur, DIF personnel restructured their program to study the effects of introducing minimally trained health and agricultural workers from local communities who were trained for relatively brief periods of time (about two months) and sent back to local communities to work on a volunteer basis. Two types of workers were trained: community health aides and community agricultural aides. The curricula for both groups included some exposure to the basic principles of public health, sanitation, nutrition, and agricultural and animal husbandry techniques, although the health workers concentrated on public health issues and the agricultural workers on agriculture. Volunteers were expected to return to their communities and take responsibility for twenty-five families.

The philosophy of development held by the DIF personnel emphasized self-sufficiency for families and communities. As a demonstration of these principles, the hacienda became more self-sufficient. Much of the food used in the large student dining hall was produced in the demonstration fields operated by DIF personnel. They also maintained a large herd of dairy cattle and a cheese-making shop, beef cattle, chickens for eggs and meat, a vegetable garden, and a bakery. Excess production from these enterprises was marketed within the valley.

Finally, the state-level Agency for Agricultural Development for the State of Mexico (DAGEM), which had been operating in the Temascalcingo area for a number of years, increased its involvement by opening an office in the municipal *cabecera* (town center) of Temascalcingo in 1977. DAGEM had been involved in a number of the development projects that have operated in the valley. DAGEM personnel had worked with Plan Lerma and Plan Maiz. A DAGEM veterinarian had been located in the hacienda for many years and had been involved in the attempt to introduce dairying into the area.

The head of the newly created DAGEM office in Temascalcingo held a different view of development. Although DAGEM had been somewhat involved in the formation of dairy cooperatives, in 1977 the director believed that the road to development for peasants was not through large projects involving abrupt change and technologizing, but through the development of locally adapted technology and small-scale, family-based enterprise. He pointed to the lack of success of large projects that have attempted to promote the formation of cooperatives, noting that they have often been co-opted by locally powerful people.

In sum, then, a number of attempts to increase the agricultural productivity of the Temascalcingo region have been made in the Valley of Temascalcingo since the redistribution of land in the mid-1930s. The projects have promoted a number of development strategies including the improvement of animal husbandry through improvement of family herds with the introduction of improved breeds of animals and the use of commercial feeds and vaccination; the improvement of maize production for home consumption and to produce a surplus for sale through the use of mechanical cultivation, chemical fertilizers and pesticides, and hybrid seed; the introduction of forage crops as cash crops; and finally, the promotion of large-scale dairying cooperatives through the promotion of forage crops, modern barns and dairying equipment, and purebred dairy cattle.

Despite this long history, development efforts in the valley have yielded little clear-cut change. Most of the programs noted above have been deemed failures, and program after program has been abandoned in disgust by change agents.

THE STUDY COMMUNITY

The community under study is located in the municipality of Temascalcingo in the Valley of Temascalcingo. Like the other barrios of Temascalcingo, this community has a Mazahua Indian heritage. Although all community members speak Spanish, many older community members speak Mazahua and remember a time when Mazahua was the language used in most homes. Younger community members no longer learn Mazahua, but the community still identifies itself as "of the Indian." About half of the approximately 250 families living in the three settlements that make up the community have access to land in the community *ejido*. The *ejido*, the school, and the church serve to tie the three settlements together. The community has a long history and existed as one of the Indian villages supplying labor to the hacienda during the colonial period. The *ejido* lands were granted in the 1930s and each of the 140 *ejidatarios* was granted 2.38 hectares of irrigated land and access to communally held hillside rain-fed agricultural land, pasture land, and forest.

Studies focusing on the impact of agricultural policy on small farmers, as translated through the development projects undertaken in the Valley of Temascalcingo, were carried out in this community in the years 1970, 1973, and 1977. The studies included an analysis of agricultural innovation and factors affecting diet.

No single development project in this community has been completely successful from the point of view of the development agents and national policy objectives. However, agricultural strategies have changed, and individual families have developed strategies that differentially emphasize subsistence production and production for exchange. Alternative agricultural strategies as well as other household variables allow families to exploit different food resources, resulting in a set of associated "nutritional strategies." Several alternative nutritional strategies are explored within the context of agricultural strategies emphasizing production for home consumption as compared to strategies with more emphasis on cash cropping.

Although there has been no monolithic adoption of any single development program in the community, the rapid succession of development efforts have left behind some change. The result is a diversification of productive techniques and crop choices. Some *ejidatarios* have taken advantage of available expertise and credit arrangements to use fertilizer, or plow with tractors, or improve their animals. DeWalt (1979) demonstrated that the adoption of introduced techniques has not been haphazard but has in fact been patterned, with some individuals adopting one set of strategies while other individuals have chosen other sets. He has called these sets of practices "agricultural adaptive strategies." Analyzing the various agricultural practices followed by a sample of sixty-two *ejidatarios* (which corresponds to the large sample used in the present study), DeWalt has been able to identify five independent agricultural strategies using a factor analytic technique.

Agricultural Strategies

The first strategy identified is "forage production." Individuals who follow this strategy have invested in the production of forage crops, partially to provide feed for their own animals, but most importantly to be used as a cash crop. The second strategy is "animal improvement." Individuals following this strategy are investing their resources in animal husbandry, vaccinating their animals, feeding them commercially produced feeds and bathing their animals. The third strategy, "tractor use," is identified by the use of tractors in cultivation. The fourth strategy, "fertilizer use," identifies people who had adopted the use of chemical fertilizers for the production of corn. A fifth strategy is followed by individuals who have not adopted any of the introduced techniques mentioned above. These people are continuing to follow a pattern of "subsistence agriculture," using the traditional methods of cultivation with emphasis on animal husbandry.

The factors defining these strategies are orthogonal (i.e., not correlated), which means that the adoption of one strategy does not imply that any other strategies are being used. Individuals who are using tractors on their fields are not necessarily using more fertilizer, and those individuals who have gone into forage crop production are generally not also adopting livestock-raising innovations. Agricultural strategies, then, are conceptually distinct and empirically independent of one another. Also, they are not mutually exclusive, and a family can be following more than one. It is possible to describe each family in terms of its degree of involvement in each of the strategies.

Most families are economically unable to participate in all programs and adopt all techniques. The result is that, for a number of different reasons, different individuals have opted to invest their resources in different strategies. Some have placed an emphasis on the improvement of their corn crop through the use of "green revolution" techniques, which include mechanization and use of chemical fertilizers. Others have adopted techniques for the improvement of animal husbandry, while still others have turned to the production of new forage crops as cash crops. Finally, some have continued to follow traditional methods of cultivating maize to meet household requirements.

There are some nonagricultural strategies being followed as well. A number of people have migrated permanently to urban areas (most notably Mexico City). They are obviously not included in this study. Some *ejidatarios,* however, migrate seasonally to the city in search of work. Others engage in wage labor when it is available. Seasonal migration and local wage labor can have an important effect on the economic adaptation of families.

The choice of agricultural strategy made by an individual or family is influenced by a complex web of factors which include ecological, economic, political, and social variables.

The production of forage crops is the most costly strategy and is at the same time the most potentially profitable. The sowing of forage crops for families with small amounts of land, however, means that a significant portion of land needs to be taken from the cultivation of staple crops. Ability to manipulate the political situation of the *ejido* and wealth are most closely associated with forage production. These two factors represent greater availability of land and capital for investment into forage as a cash crop.

Animal improvement is also an expensive strategy. It means investing in vaccines, veterinary care, and in some cases commercial foods, as well as in the animal themselves—by far the largest investment. Those who invest in animals are those who have more economic resources and who live farther from their lands. The distance from land most likely acts to discourage investment of capital in cultivation. Also, those people who spend considerable time outside the region can delegate the care of animals to other family members more easily than other agricultural tasks. The negative association of animal improvement with alcohol use reflects a common occurrence in which an individual on an alcoholic "bender" sells off animals for cash in order to continue drinking. Alcoholics tend to keep animals for only short periods of time. Women complain that their husbands during a drunken spree sometimes sell off animals that the women themselves have raised.

The use of tractors, a step towards the mechanization of agriculture, attracts both heavy users of alcohol and men who have turned to non-local strategies. Hiring a tractor and driver to do plowing releases these *ejidatarios* from having to do the cultivation themselves. Also, those who have had a greater amount of contact with change agents are more likely to use tractors. Furthermore, the use of fertilizers is not well explained. Those who see themselves as more Indian and those who are more oriented to places outside the local area are somewhat more likely to use fertilizer than others, but much of the variation in fertilizer use is left unexplained.

Finally, the last agricultural strategy—subsistence agriculture—is the oldest and is defined by the absence of innovations. Those *ejida-*

tarios least likely to continue to cultivate corn traditionally are those whose orientation is directed outside of the local area. This may seem a contradiction in that those least interested in agriculture are most likely to be investing in innovation. However, most of the introduced technologies allow for someone with sufficient capital to get some return on his land while putting in a minimal amount of personal effort.

Diet in the Research Community

Research on food use and diet was carried out in the research community during field trips in 1973 and 1977 as part of the study of agricultural change. Ethnographic information was collected to identify food sources and the resources needed to exploit alternative food sources. In addition to ethnographic information, a randomly drawn one-half sample of households with access to *ejido* land ($N = 62$) were formally interviewed in 1973. A subsample of twenty-nine households were re-interviewed in 1977.

Dietary data were collected for the sixty-two sample households in August, September, and October, 1973. A listing of foods entering the household in the preceding week and their sources was collected for each household, and twenty-four-hour recalls of household meals for the day preceding the interview were collected. The subsample of twenty-nine households were re-interviewed in September and October, 1977. Foods entering the household in the preceding week were again surveyed, and twenty-four-hour recalls of family meals were collected on three randomly drawn days for each household.

Measuring Dietary Adequacy

For this study, a combination of twenty-four-hour recalls and a "market basket" interview in which all foods entering the household and their sources were reported were used to collect dietary data. The market basket interview was used with the recall data in order to account for at least weekly cycles of food use during the research period.

The data were collected from meal makers for the sample families. Amounts of foods used during the recall days and foods acquired for the week before the household interview were estimated by the meal maker. Because of the methodological choices made, it is not possible to provide accurate figures for individuals' nutrient intakes. A series of index variables that are suggestive of adequacy and amenable to quantitative analysis was constructed. These are summarized in table 1. They include the consumption of "key foods," overall protein consumption, the proportion of protein from various sources, energy consumption from major sources, and a measure of dietary complexity.

Key foods are foods that contribute the major part of the energy, protein, and other important nutrients to the diet. For this community, they are maize, beans, milk, eggs, meat, wild greens, and purchased vegetables. Key food scores were constructed by dividing the amounts of these foods available for the household for the week by seven and then again by the number of people in the household to arrive at a daily

Table 1

Average Figures for Food Consumption Variables for 1973 and 1977

Food Variable	Full Sample 1973	1973	Subsample 1977
Maize	589.0	540.0	509.0
Beans	37.5	49.0	43.8
Sopa	—	—	15.4
Eggs	0.38	0.2	0.31
Milk consumption (ml/person/day)	156.6	86.0	104.5
Meat consumption (g/person/day)	29.1	17.0	36.0*
Use of wild greens (times/week)	1.2	1.2	1.4
Protein from major sources (g/person/day)	71.3	66.08	51.0
Protein from major vegetable sources (g/person/day)	64.3	60.58	44.3
Protein from major animal sources (g/person/day)	6.9	5.5	6.7
Protein ratio 1 (% from animal sources)	.09	.08	.13
Kcal/day from major sources	2390.0	2198.0	2063.0
Family energy-needs ratio	—	—	1.01
Family protein-needs ratio (NPU 60)	—	—	1.1
Dietary complexity score (DCS)	5.27	5.61	7.38*

*Difference significant at the .05 level using T-test for matched samples.

average availability per capita. This was done to compensate for an uneven distribution of consumption of certain foods throughout the week (most notably meat) and to correct for the size of the household. Wild green use is represented by the number of times that each family used wild greens in the week. The amount of protein provided by the foods mentioned above was calculated on a per capita basis, and several indices were constructed. The amounts of protein available from animal and vegetable sources were calculated separately. A score was calculated for the percentage of protein coming from animal sources.

For the data collected in 1977, it was possible to calculate the calories and protein available to family members from *all* foods used in the week. Also, for this year the total energy and protein requirements for each family were calculated using tables published by the World Health Association (WHO/FAO 1973). For 1977, then, ratios for the percentage of family energy and protein needs met by foods available were calculated.

A measure of dietary complexity was also constructed. All foods mentioned in recalls of family meals were summed and then divided by the number of days for which recalls were available for the family. The Dietary Complexity Score (DCS), then, is an average of the number of different foods used by a family, regardless of the amount used. Dietary complexity has been used as an index of dietary adequacy on the assumption that a more complex diet is more likely to be adequate.

The average values for the food variables are also included in table 1. On the average, the amount of energy and protein available to households met household needs. However, about half of the households failed to meet their calculated energy requirements. Maize provided, on the average, 71 percent of the energy and 65 percent of the protein available. Beans contributed about 11 percent of the protein available and foods of animal origin about 13 percent.

Nutritional Strategies

Dietary adequacy can be met in a number of ways, through a number of foods. In agrarian communities food can enter households along several paths; that is, several food sources can be exploited. Foods may be produced within households; they may be purchased; they may be gathered or hunted; they may enter households as gifts or as part of ritual (DeWalt 1981). The food use variables represent several major pathways along which foods enter households. Some of the foods are wholly purchased (meat), some may be purchased or produced within the household (maize, beans, eggs, milk), and some foods are gathered (wild greens).

The resources needed to exploit each of these potential paths are somewhat different. The ability to purchase foods is related to the ability to generate cash income; the use of home produced foods to the availability of land, crop choices, labor allocation, and use of inputs. The use of wild foods may be related to the location of the household with respect to wild food resources and the availability of household labor to exploit them. Finally, the degree to which food is received as gifts or through ritual exchange may be a function of the social ties enjoyed by a household and the involvement of household members in community life. The relatively complex nature of the resulting nutritional system of agrarian communities means that the nutritional consequences of agricultural change may be correspondingly complex.

Increases in cash income, the implicit goal of many agricultural development projects and the explicit goal of those that promote cash cropping, can be expected to most dramatically affect the use of those foods that are purchased. Use of home-produced foods may be unaffected, or negatively affected, by the generation of income. An analysis of the effects of increasing income on the food use of households in this community (DeWalt 1983a) has shown a linear relationship between income and the consumption of meat and milk, foods purchased by most households; and a weaker relationship with the consumption of eggs, a food that is purchased by some households and produced by others. The dietary complexity score was also significantly related to differences in wealth. The use of basic staples, such as maize and beans, wild foods, and the degree to which families were able to meet their protein and energy requirements were not linearly related to wealth. It was concluded that although the very poorest families had inadequate diets as measured by the amount of energy available, after a certain point increasing wealth resulted in a different diet, but not necessarily a better diet.

Agricultural Strategies and Food Use

Each of the agricultural strategies has potential effects on diet. Some of these are direct consequences of the crop choices themselves, affecting the production of specific food items. Other consequences are indirect in that they affect the generation of cash and hence the ability of a household to purchase food items. In this section I will examine each strategy in terms of its potential effects on diet and examine the relationships between agricultural strategy and food use in the data from the study community for 1973.

It was expected that the agricultural strategies adopted by the families would have an impact on households' diets that was more complex than a direct effect as a result of income generation. To examine the relationships between the choice of agricultural strategy and food use strategy, correlation coefficients were calculated.

The correlation coefficients between the agricultural strategies and the food use variables for 1973 can be found in table 2. Because both the choice of agricultural strategy followed and some aspects of food use are affected by economic standing, the correlations in table 2 are first-order partial correlations in which economic standing is controlled for statistically.

Forage production. Forage, as it was cultivated in 1973, was viewed as a cash crop. Most forage was sold in local markets. Some families, who were also investing in the animal improvement strategy, used some of their forage production as feed for their own animals, but these were few in number. For successful cultivation, forage crops need good soil and frequent irrigation. Forage was to grow on the best irrigated land, on the valley floor. In order to grow forage crops, then, an *ejidatario* had to take some part of the best maize-growing land out of maize production and allocate it to forage. In 1977, the amount of maize produced was a major determinant of the adequacy of protein and energy provided by the diet. The shift to production of a forage crop may have had a detrimental effect on diet if the amount of cash generated was not adequate to replace the lost produced foods with purchased foods. I expected, then, that adoption of forage production would be negatively related to use of maize and beans and positively related to use of purchased foods.

When the relationships between investment in forage production and food use patterns are viewed, however, there are no clear-cut relationships either negatively with maize and legume consumption or positively with the use of specific purchased foods. A relationship between forage production and the overall use of foods of animal origin

Table 2
First-Order Partial Correlations of Agricultural Strategies with Food Use, Controlling for Wealth, 1973

Food Consumption Variable	Agricultural Strategies				
	Forage Production	Tractor Use	Fertilizer Use	Livestock Improvement	Subsistence Agriculture
Maize consumption	-.01	-.07	.16	-.23*	.09
Bean consumption	-.01	-.07	-.03	.11	.00
Meat consumption	.07	.33*	.20	.07	-.34*
Milk consumption	.00	-.09	.02	.38*	-.16
Egg consumption	.05	.00	-.16	-.02	.06
Protein from vegetable sources	-.05	-.09	.07	-.10	.09
Protein from animal sources	.46*	-.07	-.10	.37*	-.34*
Total protein	-.08	-.06	.06	-.13	.11
Protein from animal sources/total protein	.67**	.01	-.08	.48**	-.56**
Wild green consumption	.13	.11	-.04	-.02	-.09
Dietary complexity	-.03	.25*	-.07	.33*	-.27*

*$p < .05$
**$p < .01$

does appear, suggesting that forage production affects the use of foods of animal origin positively. That is, the total amount of use is higher for households investing in forage production. The use of single foods is not significantly greater in this group, though.

In 1977 the amount of maize produced was associated with maize consumption. In that year more land was dedicated to forage production and had a more clear-cut relationship with food use. In table 3, correlations between the amount of land planted in maize and the percentage of land planted in forage crops and the food use variables for 1977 are presented. The percentage of land in forage crops is negatively related to the use of maize, beans, and wild greens, but these relationships are not statistically significant. Because economic status co-varies with both forage production and food use, I have also calculated the first-order partial coefficients controlling for wealth for these variables in 1977. These can also be found in table 3. Controlling for economic status does have some effect on the correlations. The correlations between the amount of land planted in corn and the consumption of meat and the energy needs ratio become lower and lose statistical significance. Those who plant more maize consume more milk and have a more complex diet. On the other hand, when all the families in the subsample are considered, the percentage of land in forage crops has a negative effect on the energy and protein needs ratios, and the amount of land planted in corn has a positive effect, although these relationships are not statistically significant.

Tractor and fertilizer usage. The use of tractors and fertilizer are both aspects of "green revolution" technology. They were introduced by development agents in order to improve maize production. The use of tractors in plowing has been adopted primarily by people who are less interested in farming. The cost of plowing with a tractor is no more expensive for a family without a team of draft animals than the cost of renting a team. The application of fertilizer to maize crops does require an extra outlay of cash. In 1973, however, there was credit available to purchase fertilizer. The use of fertilizer and tractors does correlate with maize production but the correlation coefficients are not very high. Maize production is more closely related to the quality and quantity of the land held by the *ejidatario,* which is in turn related to the political power exerted by the individual in *ejido* affairs (DeWalt 1979). Because the use of tractors is associated with an orientation

Table 3

Correlations of the Amount of Land in Maize and Percentage of Land
in Forage with Food Use, 1977

Food Use Variable	Zero Order Correlations		First-Order Partial Correlations Controlling for Wealth	
	% Land in Forage	Amt. of Land in Maize	% Land in Forage	Amt. of Land in Maize
Maize consumption	−.19	.03	−.23	.01
Bean consumption	−.29	.30	−.30	.31
Milk consumption	.02	.35*	.01	.37*
Meat consumption	.17	.42*	−.02	.33
Egg consumption	.18	−.21	.11	−.29
Wild greens	−.30	.14	−.31	.15
DCS	−.06	.43*	−.15	.40*
Energy-needs ratio	−.19	.40*	−.31	.35
Protein-needs ratio	−.06	.33	−.21	.24

*$p < .05$

towards pursuits other than local agriculture, people who use tractors
may also be using cash generated through wage labor to purchase a
more complex diet.

When the use of these technologies is viewed in terms of food use,
the adoption of innovations designed to improve maize production appears to have little effect. There are no significant correlations between
fertilizer use and food use. The use of tractors is associated with the
consumption of meat and, more weakly, with the complexity of the
diet. Tractor use is associated with increased corn production (but not
consumption), and it may be that cash generated from the sale of maize
is used to purchase a slightly more varied diet.

Livestock improvement. Animal husbandry is a relatively expensive
strategy for investment. However, improvement of livestock raising
does not necessarily require that land be taken from the production of
staple crops (although livestock improvement is somewhat related to
forage production). It is also a venture for which the labor required,

mainly pasturing the animals, can be allocated to relatively unskilled members of the family. For this reason, investment in improved animal husbandry is a strategy which is frequently followed by *ejidatarios* who spend considerable time working in urban areas. Among the animals kept, the most important and most common animal is the cow. The cows kept are of a local breed (*criollo*). Development agents have complained in the past that the *criollo* breed is an inferior milker and that small-scale, family-based cattle keeping in which the cattle are fed primarily through grazing is an inefficient way of producing milk. As noted above, the most recent development programs in the region have stressed large-scale dairying efforts using purebred cattle fed a blend of high-grade forage and commercial feeds. The introduction of large-scale dairying enterprises has contributed little to the availability of milk in the valley, however. Most of the milk consumed and sold is produced by households with small numbers of animals. Households that have invested time and other resources into improving their backyard herds would likely be able to consume more dairy products and to enjoy the benefits of increased income as a result of the sale of milk and milk products. In fact, animal improvement is the strategy with the strongest positive impact on food use.

Subsistence maize production. Some families have continued to plant primarily maize without mechanization and fertilizer. Those following the strategy of subsistence maize cultivation also tend to be poorer and to identify more strongly with the community's Indian heritage. It was expected that families that have not adopted any alternative strategy would rely more heavily on staple food items and less on purchased foods. However, there is no relationship between subsistence agriculture and the use of maize, beans, or wild greens. There are significant negative correlations with the consumption of meat and animal products, although not with overall protein consumption. In looking at the overall patterning of association between agricultural strategies and diet, the most striking thing is the relative lack of association. None of the strategies is associated either positively or negatively with the overall protein content of the diet, although forage production and animal improvement are associated with the quality of the protein available. To the extent to which dietary complexity reflects dietary quality, families who keep animals and invest in their care are more likely to have a better overall diet. To a lesser extent, families who use tractors also have a somewhat better diet. It appears that a gradual shift in recent years from subsistence maize cultivation to the cultivation of forage crops has not had a dramatic effect on diet. On the other hand, programs to introduce improved maize cultivation have had even less effect. In 1973 at least, those who were following an agricultural strategy which included an emphasis on small-scale animal keeping with the inclusion of one or two dairy cattle producing for home consumption had a greater dietary advantage. In 1973 maize production was not significantly related to nutritional status, but in 1977, when a greater number of families had dedicated some land to the cultivation of forage crops, differentials in maize production were related to dietary adequacy as measured by the degree to which family needs for energy and protein were met.

Conversations with development agents working in communities which had already entered into a cooperative dairying enterprise suggested that the cooperatives were not able to produce a profit and any economic benefits would have been siphoned off to pay for the enormous debt incurred by the *ejido* in the construction of the stable facilities and the purchase of quality dairy cattle. Even in theoretical terms, then, it seems that the dairying project would have been unlikely to produce enough revenue to offset the loss of subsistence foods which would have been grown on the land now devoted to forage production.

Development efforts in the area do not seem to have had an important impact on poor diet and nutrition in the community. As has been pointed out, those who have benefited most from development efforts have been those who were more economically well off to begin with. The agricultural strategies which have the greatest impact on diet are those which selectively use parts of modern technology within a traditional subsistence framework. The animal improvement strategy, in which some aspects of improved animal husbandry are incorporated into the maintenance of a small dairy herd for home use, has the greatest impact on diet within the community.

It is the secondary benefits of the development process that seem to have had the greatest impact on diet. When the dietary patterns of families studied in both 1973 and 1977 are compared for the two years, a change can be seen (table 1). However, this change in diet seems to be most clearly related to the effects of an increase in employment among the families of this community. The increase in employment is attributable to construction work which was done on the river in 1977. For six months or so before my fieldwork began in 1977, construction crews had been hiring local men to do unskilled labor connected with the construction of levees on the river to further control flooding. Hence, the number of persons in sample households employed in wage work almost doubled between 1973 and 1977. This results in an increase in average dietary complexity and the use of animal products with a related fall in the use of maize and beans. Unfortunately, the increase in labor opportunities was to be temporary. The best estimate of the companies overseeing the work was that the project would be finished by early 1978. The long-term effects of this factor on diet will probably be minimal, although only further research in the community will tell.

SUGGESTED ALTERNATIVE POLICIES

The data and analyses of the nutritional system in this agricultural community in rural Mexico suggest several possible approaches to nutritional improvement, or at least maintenance of the status quo. The encouragement of self-sufficiency through the development of small-family livestock keeping, cultivation of sufficient legumes to meet household needs, and possibly the encouragement of small horticultural crops would seem to have beneficial effects on families' diets. The land base available does not seem to be sufficiently large that the income generated through the cultivation of forage crops on an individual level would make up for the loss of subsistence crops. Experience in other communities further suggests that cooperative ventures growing forage crops are faced with the same problem. The creation of employment opportunities would likely improve the nutritional status as well as the overall economic standing of people in the community. In fact, the people of this community themselves feel that their greatest lack is sufficient wage labor employment opportunities.

The situation found in the study community parallels the consequences of the development effort in Mexico on a national level. As a result of substantial investment in agricultural research, irrigation facilities, credit, and subsidization of most agricultural inputs, Mexico's production of maize, wheat, and sorghum increased eightfold between

1940 and 1979. During this same time period, population only tripled (DeWalt 1985). Despite the substantial growth of food production, the nutritional status of large parts of the Mexican population has remained poor, with many children suffering mild to moderate malnutrition (Chavez 1974, 1982; Perez Hidalgo 1976; Dewey 1983).

The problem is that the increased production of grains is not going to improve the diet of the estimated nineteen million Mexicans whose daily calorie and protein intake is below that required for physical well-being (Redclift 1981). All of the sorghum and an estimated 13 percent of the maize in Mexico are being used to feed animals to satisfy the growing demand for meat among the affluent sectors of the population. The same shifts that I have identified in the study community are occurring on a national level. As segments of the population obtain the economic resources to do so, they shift to more affluent diets containing more meat, replace maize with wheat products, and use more processed foods. These diets are not necessarily more adequate—they are only more costly. At the same time, the small-farm families who have contributed in part to increased productivity remain economically and nutritionally marginal.

Mental Health Services in Micronesia: A Case of Superficial Development

Albert B. Robillard

A leading piece in the United States development effort in the Trust Territory of the Pacific Islands has been health services. Soon after the creation of a Territorial Bureau of Health, mental health services were added to upgrade the existing services. The expatriate mental health professionals hired to implement the new service proclaimed that the Micronesian islanders of the territory were without a sense of psychology or introspection; indigenous islanders hired to assist the Western mental health professionals were in immediate need of formal instruction in psychology. Psychological training and service development efforts of the new Division of Mental Health for the Territory were soon confounded, however, by structural features of Micronesian cultural, social, and political organization. An evaluation of the eleven major mental health services training and development programs in the territory found that they failed to establish stable and appropriate mental health services. This paper discusses the policy issues involved in the failure of mental health services and asks, "What explains the structural relationships, in the face of successive failure, between the advocacy and cycles of development efforts and the clear absence of compatibility of the programs developed with local cultural and political organization?" By way of conclusion, a theory of interorganizational linkages is recommended to ensure a policy and implementation interface between Western mental health constructs and Micronesian phenomenology.

FROM ASCRIPTIVE HIERARCHY TO INSTITUTIONS OF INDIVIDUALISM

When President Kennedy dispatched Professor Anthony Solomon and a host of technical experts in July of 1963 (Nevin 1977:125) to evaluate the circumstances of the people living in the Trust Territory of the Pacific Islands—an administrative mandate assigned to the United States by the United Nations—the evaluation group perceived and reported Pacific Islanders living in a historical vacuum. They reported that the people were greatly affected by the movements of men and material of the Second World War, but since that time they have been living in a suspended state, somewhere between traditional political orders and surface changes effected by a relatively passive colonial administration run by the United States Navy and the Department of Interior (Hanlon and Eperiam 1983:85). It was clear that the people occupying two thousand islands of Micronesia were not synchronized with the worldwide penetration of the industrialized world political economies to the lesser developed countries. It was even problematic whether Micronesia could be placed parallel to any set of developing Third World nations, as Micronesia had barely moved along any developmental path, except perhaps backward, since the cessation of World War II (Fischer and Fischer 1957:59). What had once been a highly commodity-oriented local economy under Japanese administration in the early forties had now reverted to a subsistence economy based on local agriculture and fishing (Schwalbenberg 1984:2–10).

The material conditions of government and agriculture had rapidly declined after wartime seizure of the islands from the Japanese. Japan had populated the islands with large numbers of its own workers, utilizing the islands for intensive agriculture, fishing, and mining, as well as for strategically occupying a large portion of the western Pacific (Hanlon and Eperiam 1983:84). The Japanese had established a school system, electrification (sometimes with hydroelectric power), paved roads, harbors and docks, mercantile establishments, shipping routes, and radio communication. The capital improvements infrastructure established by the Japanese was destroyed or left in a state of disrepair with the onset of American administration in 1945. The United States Department of Defense kept the entire area under security wraps for the first twenty years of administration. Access to the area was limited to those with clearance from the Chief of U.S. Naval Operations.

Japan had administered the islands comprising the territory after taking them from Germany during the First World War in 1914. Germany held the islands from 1899, purchasing them from Spain at the end of the Spanish-American War (Fischer and Fischer 1957:47; Hezel 1984:20). The islands were of value to Germany for copra, for trading opportunities for a handful of Oceania-based German merchants, and for phosphate in Palau and Mauru (Hezel 1984:21). With the exception of the Christianization interests of Catholic missionaries, Spain had had comparatively little interest in the aggregated 708 square miles of land that compose what is now the Trust Territory. Spain had held formal claim to the area from 1885 to 1914.

The conditions of the United Nations trusteeship mandate were to develop the islands to the point that the indigenous peoples would independently decide upon and execute their political futures. Development was expected in terms of education and the creation of an infrastructure compatible with the economic and social participation in the world political economy, the hope or unstated background premise, perhaps, being that such participation would acquire and equitably distribute a resource base that would create pluralistic structures of social democracy.

A visit, in 1961, to the Trust Territory by a United Nations delegation charged with oversight of UN-mandated trust territories and the group's subsequent report delivered a stinging rebuke to America's well-developed self-image as a leader for self-determination and social-economic development (Hanlon and Eperium 1983:86). The UN group, composed in part by prominent Third World political leaders, found the Micronesian inhabitants of the Trust Territory kept in isolation to meet American security interests and, in such a condition, retained the hierarchically arranged ascriptive social structures— structures by which subsistence agricultural and fishing societies had been historically built (Alkire 1972; Schwalbenberg 1984:2–10). The hierarchies were many, loosely joined to one another, each having an independent base of power, often related to the natural ecology and isolation of each island group. These societies formed fragmented collectivities, organized around trade and tribute relations to stronger groups; but there was relatively little in the way of central direction across island groups. The everyday affairs of each were self-contained (Alkire 1972). Within each of these island societies there was little in the way of movement toward the acquisition of capital appreciation resources which would permit significant Micronesian participation in the market economies of the world.

The first task the Kennedy Administration saw for itself was to develop in Micronesia the social institutions of an American-style democratic pluralism—what Aaron Wildavsky, characterizing the United States, calls "a compromise between economic individualism, political egalitarianism and social hierarchy" (1982:4)—and to thereby bind by preference the inhabitants of the Trust Territory to affiliation with the United States. The second objective was to maintain the strategic importance of the territory, the subject of National Security Council Memoranda (Nevin 1977). Primary channels of achieving both ends were education, health development, and the creation of central state government bureaucracies, one for each political district, based on universalistic values for achievement, individualism and egalitarianism, and popular representative governments. Even with the death of President Kennedy, the New Frontier style of development by projection of American social institutions continued with massive increases in numbers of American teachers, Peace Corps workers, and expatriate American technical consultants and administrators.

A key, if totally unexamined, element in the development of institutions of pluralistic individualism was the creation and maintenance of Western standards of health and health services. Health services, seemingly innocuous on the surface, substantively altered the structure of traditional ascriptive societies. First, health services in Micronesia would become universally available, thereby attenuating dependency and accompanying definitions of action for lower social castes and classes of people. Universal health care services alter the hierarchical control of health resources (traditional medicine practitioners, medications, and even nutrition), resources which heretofore were consonant with traditional ascriptive political economies. Second, universal health care, based upon hypothetico-deductive science, a form of reason external to indigenous resources, offers explanations and therapeutic guidance which, again, are asynchronous with ascriptively distributed knowledge about sickness, health, and the causes of each. Allopathic medicine is universalistic in application, treating all members of the society in the same fashion, subject to the same laws of pathophysiology. Third, health care services offer employment based upon achieved merit. This norm, though frequently recognized in the breach, is but another institution in creating a society of individuals, each an independent unit capable of acquiring and controlling resources. This is very different than other formulations of what it means to be human, conceptions, such as in Yap, where people are thought to be extensions of ancestral lands (Labby 1976:16), not free individuals acquiring and disposing of goods according to individuals needs. Fourth, by creating a health services system which is universally accessible and administered by the central state, spanning all divisions of the society, the institutions of individualism are infused across the entire social fabric. Health care, thus administered, is isomorphic with the creation, as one system, of cultural definition principles and perceiving subjects of individualism (Archibald 1978:2–13).

The point here is to recognize that the establishment of universalistic health care services carries with it fundamentally specific background definitions of the person, an entity universally assessed on the basis of individual conditions and attainments. The fact that American health development planners might have failed to explicitly recognize the metaphysical premises of health care and the impact that such health care would have upon traditional ascriptive Oceanic political economies is less an absence of evidence of the cultural impact upon Micronesians of American-style health care than it is, perhaps, of the unexamined social origin of those health development plans.

Another part of development for the Trust Territory was mandatory and universal education, pedagogy structurally mirroring American education, with the ultimate objective for the student being college entrance and/or the subsequent acquisition of salaried employment (Hezel 1982: 19–30; Nevin 1977). As with medicine, the content of education and the subjects to be educated are treated with universalistic criteria, the bedrock of individualism. The topics of education are open to any perceiving subject, accessible to anyone. In turn, each perceiving subject possesses an equivalent ability to apprehend.

Election to government positions by universal suffrage and employment based upon achieved merit are equally obvious sources of generating a society dependent upon the institution of individualism, the American vision of development, a sight equally embedded in most versions of development. Even the United Nations critique of American development efforts in Micronesia was driven from premises of developing individuals for participation in a society of individual acquisition and disposition, the world economy. Micronesians of the Trust Territory were perceived as undeveloped precisely because they did not possess social institutions for participation in the world economy, an economy based upon a distinct technostructure of institutional fabric (Wallerstein 1979:23).

BUREAU OF HEALTH SERVICES AND THE IMAGE OF UPGRADING: AN EXAMPLE OF INSTITUTIONAL REPLICATION

With the idea of creating the technostructure of Western-style health care and, implicitly, the broader institutional fabric which created and supports American-style health care, the U.S. Department of Interior, upon taking up administration of the Trust Territory from the navy in 1951, established the Trust Territory Bureau of Health Services. The bureau, under the high commissioner of the Trust Territory, developed health care services for each of the then subadministrative districts of the territory: the Marshall Islands, Ponape-Kosrae, Truk, Yap, Palau, and the Northern Marianas. Health services for each of the island groups or districts were coordinated from the bureau's central headquarters on the island of Saipan in the Northern Marianas. Individual-island group health services were housed in hospitals located in the population centers of each district. Indigenous Micronesians were selected and sent to the Fiji Medical Officer (M.O.) training program, at what is now the medical school of the University of the South Pacific. The medical officers or M.O.'s quickly replaced expatriate U.S. civilian and navy physicians. In some districts, however, expatriate contract or National Health Service Corps physicians continued and still serve patient care roles. Micronesian M.O.'s are now, though, the senior management of the various health services. With the anticipated breakup of the Trust Territory into three independent nation-states and one commonwealth of the United States, the territory Bureau of Health Services will dissolve, each nation and the Commonwealth of the Northern Marianas undertaking administration of its health services.

The Bureau of Health Services has over the last several years reduced its functions to coordination of planning and bulk purchasing.

At the height of its direct management role, the Bureau of Health Services established and administered a Division of Mental Health. Records of the Bureau of Health Services date the beginning of the division in 1969 (Gellen 1970). An initial project of the division was a mental health training program for Micronesian health services. The program was implemented at the hospital on Saipan. The trainees were police, Head Start teachers and village commissioners (Gellen 1970). This was to be the first of at least eleven mental health service training programs to be held for Micronesians over the next thirteen years (appendix).

Training indigenous personnel in mental health services skills was of critical importance in a geographic area containing at least nine major language groups, with many subdialects. Micronesian staff would assist the one bureau psychiatrist on Saipan, providing the only link between the psychiatrist and the linguistic, cultural, and social world of the patients. Mental health trainees were and continue to be the conduit for implementing psychiatric and psychological services.

What led to creation of the Division of Mental Health? It is very tempting to say that perception of need and other motives for establishing a specialized division of mental health services were unrelated to empirical investigations of the mental health status of Micronesians. But, then, the credibility of this kind of assertion rests on the assumption that the question of mental health service needs of a population is answered by empirical investigation of the population. There are, at least in practice, other ways of establishing services needs. Lawrence Wilson, M.D., onetime director of the Division of Mental Health, wrote: "In the late 1960's U.S. Federal grant money became available to upgrade health services and some specific funds were allocated to develop a mental health program. A psychiatrist was recruited from the U.S. and later a psychologist was added." (Wilson 1981:163). At first blush, the reader might want to say that "upgrading" is not generated by an analysis of Micronesian mental health phenomena, the analysis of which indicates the need for and direction of mental health services. But if we stop for a moment to consider medicine as a social institution which, in its collective imagery of man, provides a comprehensive a priori definition of man and needs, we see that the object of observation is medicine, not Micronesian life. If the basic parameters of man are given in terms of medicine, then we may look to the panoply of *services* of medicine to decide what is missing and needed in Micronesia.

The process of finding empirical or experiential justification for the elaboration of human services, by comparing the present state of services to more highly developed levels of service elsewhere, is not unique to mental health services in Micronesia. It was the basis for almost every piece of legislatively mandated human services of the 1960s and 1970s in the Trust Territory. In one of the youngest populations in the world, with a median age of 16.2 (Trust Territory of the Pacific Islands 1980:57), there exists in each district a gerontology program, complete with an "aging nurse," and trucks and boats exclusively for the use of gerontological services staff. In the Trust Territory, more than 72 percent of the people are under thirty years old. Moreover, older people are respected, cared for at home within the context of large extended families. The Trust Territory also has Head Start, as well as child and maternal health and nutrition programs, all administered by the same U.S. agencies in charge of programs by the same name in the United States.

As with mental health, the other programs were not preceded by intense, empirical service needs research. The prior existence of the service programs on the U.S. mainland and the strong definitions of human behavior and needs carried with them, as well as (no doubt) the political, professional, and personal interests served through the acquisition and administration of such programs, are the principles which organized the perception of need. Upgrades and needed programs were based upon the generalized conditions and needs of human behavior implied by the existence of programs elsewhere.

To this day there is no independent epidemiological research on mental health in the Trust Territory of the Pacific Islands. Yet there have been abundant congressional testimony, legislation, and grant applications arguing for supplying unmet Micronesian mental health care needs. The arguments find their rationality on the basis of comparing Micronesian health care to the edifice of medical care found on the U.S. mainland and upon anecdotal accounts of Micronesian mental health problems. The stories of mental health problems—invariably true, but not generated by a sampling design—appear to confirm arguments for service needs when it is pointed out that the American modalities of care for the problem reported are not found in Micronesia. Further, while a Division of Mental Health has been created, there has been scant attention paid to whether the services of the division statistically correspond to the mental health needs of the area (Robillard 1984). The empirical object of observation, comparison, and that which motivates upgrades and completions of care within the Bureau of Health Services—as in the case of the Division of Mental Health—are the social institutions of medicine in the United States, not the health profile of Micronesia.

AN UPGRADE MEETS MICRONESIAN SOCIAL AND CULTURAL ORGANIZATION

The creation of mental health services in the Trust Territory took two avenues. The first was the establishment of the Division of Mental Health within the Bureau of Health Services on Saipan. The second, necessitated for reasons discussed above, was the selection and training of mental health coordinators, individuals who would be the operational conduit of the services in each local hospital. The coordinators worked under the direction of both their immediate hospital-based medical officer supervisors and the Saipan-based, expatriate director of the Division of Mental Health. Recruitment and training of indigenous mental health service personnel, as witnessed in the initial work of the division and thereafter, became a paramount focus of the division. Problems emerged quickly, problems for which solutions have yet to be found.

Dr. Lawrence Wilson (1981), the only psychiatrist of the four successive directors of the Division of Mental Health to publish on the structure and performance of the division, summed up the problems perceived by the various training efforts. First, he found that previous training of Micronesian paraprofessionals "had nothing of substance from which further training as a mental health paraprofessional could be built. And since most Micronesian cultures tend not to be psychologically minded or introspective this was a significant problem to be overcome. A detailed course on normal personality development was developed for the mental health coordinators (and selected school teachers) to partially remedy this problem" (1981:168).

Second, he found that "although the psychiatrist in Saipan was their "boss" (since he controlled their salary), the mental health coordinators' day-to-day work was in reality much more influenced by local island political alliances, clan or caste rivalries, family status and hospital politics. These immediate factors had far more impact on the coordinators' daily job functioning than did the psychiatrist who was sometimes several thousand miles away" (1981:168). Wilson states that counselors were often shifted to emergency room duties, night coverage, or to TB clinics, the strong message being given through these assignments that mental health was a low priority, that acute curative medicine was to take precedence (Wilson 1981:168).

Third, Wilson reports of Micronesian medical officers that "even some of those doctors assigned to be 'in charge of' psychiatry for their hospital were disinterested or uninvolved" (1981:169). However, at the same time he found Micronesian medical officers' good will essential and always in need of regeneration, lest they "sabotage the coordinator's role and work." The medical officer, he reports, would feel slighted if he were not kept fully informed; he would feel "belittled by the act that the highly trained American specialist was spending so much time with the mental health coordinators who had, in local eyes, much lower professional prestige and age-related status" (1981:169).

It is apparent from Wilson's assessment that Micronesian society and culture was perceived to be deficient in knowledge about psychological man. Wilson states that the society is not psychologically or introspectively minded. The remedy to this missing piece of essential information—knowledge which will, once possessed, fill out the imagery of man—was a training course, an education to eradicate the ignorance of Micronesians about the character of man. What is disturbing about these assertions is that no evidence is marshalled to ground characterizations of Micronesians as peoples without psychology. There is no doubt that most Micronesians do not have ready command of the principles of psychology as taught in American universities. But there is every reason to believe, just from everyday conversations and from formal ethnopsychological studies, that Micronesian cultures have detailed and ordered explanations of behavior (Lutz 1985). Many of these explanations do not correspond to the cultural structure of Eastern psychology. They are what psychology and psychiatry label folk beliefs. When incorporated into intervention strategies, they are called ethnomedicine.

The replacement of indigenous explanatory systems of behavior with modern Western psychologies apparently issues not from a detailed investigation of the local psychologies or from a reading of anthropological literature reporting the structure and function of indigenous personality and other social forms (e.g., the family, clan, island group). There is no evidence in the published and unpublished record of the Division of Mental Health, or subsequent mental health services development projects, of consulting the anthropological literature on Micronesia. Citations or textual references to the substantial amount of Micronesian study literature cannot be found. The replacement is by administrative fiat to replicate the imagery of man found in the lore and reason of Western professional psychology and psychiatry.

It is easy to see that the replacement of indigenous psychologies of Micronesians with professional Western versions of man are both a misunderstanding of the analytic structure of social science and a structured interest of professional mental health service organizations. Instead of looking to and examining Micronesian psychologies, Western psychology, the product of a distinct social context, is made a universal. In this position, Western psychology is both the method and subject of description. The projection of Western man as a universal is, at the same time, an efficient utilization of the resources and repertoires of existing Western mental health programs. Nothing new need be added. The short-term return is much greater by using existing technology. What may not be so evident is the fact that the man of Western psychology, the capsulized individual, the egalitarian subject, is totally of a piece with "the development" of Micronesia, the creation of individual participants, the ratios of labor force participation in a society in the exchange activities of the world money economy. Western psychology is required for the practice of clinical work but, at a more basic level, is a prior condition to conceiving of and accounting for the creation of a society of universally equivalent subjects, the mass society within which Western notions of development comprise a rational construct. It is in such a society that individual growth and mobility are the signposts of progress.

The next roadblock encountered by Dr. Wilson, also reported in other training programs (Robillard 1984; Tsuda 1984), is the influence of indigenous hierarchies, traditional and bureaucratic. Wilson reports that his authority was superseded by circumstances of "local island political alliances, clan or caste rivalries, family status and hospital politics." Futhermore, he reported that the indigenous medical officers were sensitive to his dealing directly with lower-status mental health counselors; medical officers had to be kept up-to-date on all activities, lest they feel offended. The phenomenon of hierarchy and how it relates to the generation and control of the health care services in Micronesia is one consistently encountered, though never fully described, in the record of Micronesian mental health development. Perhaps the inability to fully come to grips with the phenomenon is related to an intellectual incapacity of Americans to explicitly acknowledge a world in which inherited social status (caste, class, title, island of origin) is the most concrete of realities, a division irrepressibly embedded in every aspect of social life. While Americans have and must deal in their everyday lives with hierarchy, some of it ascribed, it is a driving myth of American thought that the individual is supreme, and individualism the natural state of man.

The lack of seriousness with which the developers of mental health services took indigenous hierarchy is evidenced by the fact that social class is directly described but once in the corpus of papers and reports on the development of mental health services in the Trust Territory. Attention to how indigenous hierarchies are structured and affect the capacity of Micronesian mental health services only comes after the implementation of eleven training programs, all of which were seriously co-opted by indigenous hierarchies. It is as if class or social status is not recognizable within the rhetoric of program development and education. Yet, as the only retrospective evaluation of mental health services development to date has described (Robillard 1984), in all but one island area the mental health counselors/coordinators were recruited from among outer islanders and lower-caste or untitled people. This is in cultures where class and caste distinctions are omnipresent. Further, it was found that caste, class, island, and language differences were the most prevalent obstacles for the mental health counselor, both in acquiring the resources and organizational mandate to see mental health patients and in the conduct of direct patient-care services.

Being of lower social status put the counselors at a disadvantage in interacting with patients, as well as in their capacity to become a stable set of mental health care providers. Because of low social status, the counselors were subject to being reassigned to other services, sometimes on an ad hoc basis and other times permanently. At least two counselors, both in situations where they were the only counselors for their islands, were assigned to the position of the national hypertension control officer. These assignments superseded the mental health assignments in terms of time and resources. Both individuals were expected to retain their mental health care responsibilities concurrently with their hypertension control duties. As Dr. Wilson has described, the mental health counselor is subject to the priorities of the local medical, political, and traditional hierarchies, whether in the conduct of patient care or in obtaining management recognition to conduct mental health care duties in the hospital.

A third trouble encountered by Wilson and his colleagues in mental health services development was the absence of interest in mental health by Micronesian medical officers, even among those assigned to be in charge of mental health. The consequence of the disinterest is related to the management role of the medical officers; disinterest was perceived as leading to the reassignment of mental health personnel to other duties. Mental health personnel were frequently reassigned from mental health to other services, most often acute curative care services. Medical officers were also found to be uninvolved, meaning that they did not talk about or engage in direct mental health services. They did not provide a social milieu for others to work in the area and by action and inaction relegated mental health services to a low priority.

The absence of interest and involvement is related to the assertion that Micronesians are not psychologically or introspectively minded. There is no doubt, from the reports of the eleven training programs, that Western professional psychology and psychiatry do not correspond to work organization and/or other pursuits of Micronesian medical officers. We must raise the question again, however, if it is not going a little far, if not being altogether ethnocentrically judgmental, to say that Micronesian medical officers are uninterested in mental health. Is it really possible for anyone to operate without very elaborate interpretative theories of mental health and behavior, theories which are the basis for attributing meaning to behavior, from conversational encounters to the collective rationality of large institutions? Might it be that Western psychology is uninteresting because it has not presented itself in terms of a cogent interpretation of Micronesian experience? In all of the eleven training programs, psychology was taught as basic principles by people without intimate knowledge of Micronesian cultures or languages, all illustrations having to come, then, from American experiences. Therefore, psychology was not presented as an abstraction of Micronesian experience, but as a concrete reality, one without roots in Micronesian experience.

CeCilia R. Cooper (n.d.a), a colleague of Dr. Wilson, wrote a paper entitled "Some Belated Hindsights of a Western Trainer." The paper is a reflection upon her work with Dr. Wilson in training indigenous mental health coordinators in the Trust Territory. She, like Wilson and others, was frustrated by the meager impact of the training programs. She was also concerned about the effects of the training upon the trainees, some of whom suffered, she felt, because of the training. She attempted to explain the limited services impact and pathological effects of the training upon trainees by linking aspects of Micronesian social and cultural organization to the training. She examined the community and family context of the trainees, looking at how training—the introduction of new ideas and aspirations—was at the same time a perturbation of how superiors, colleagues, family, and community perceived or treated the trainee. Reactions to the trainees, given the kind of changes being introduced and the method of introduction, could be ngative or positive. In every case, she observed, there was extreme risk for negative feedback. Mental health training transpired in a rich context, the social and cultural location of the trainee. Just the act of attendance of the training program could produce new expectations of the trainee, from both maternal and paternal sides of the extended family, which acted to curb strenuous expressions of the kind of leadership being espoused by the training. The individual who acted boldly and independently in creating a mental health service, aside from encountering the other problems set off in the ascendant hospital hierarchy, would at the same time create expectations in his family of greater material wealth and position, something relatives would call upon, something which the trainee—in a society where shame is very important—could not deliver, given the fact that the training did not provide increased standing in the hospital-based power system, nor even an increase in pay.

The contribution of Dr. Cooper lies in pointing out that development—in this case, mental health services—occurs in a context, an intersection of personal history and cultural and social structure, and that context frequently is at odds with both the ends and the means of mental health services development schemes. Power, or hierarchically arranged access to resources, however, is missing in the explanatory model, a cognitive-cultural model, advanced by Dr. Cooper. Cultural constraints upon the trainees such as family and community expectations are recognized, but it is either assumed that the circumstance of the trainees was universal among Micronesians or stratificational processes are not relevant. In any case, the class, caste, or island origin status designations of the trainees are not recognized in Cooper's analysis, thereby leaving out a critical ordering process. It is the hierarchical ordering process, the culture upon which it is based—creating subjects and objects as an integrated network—which selects trainees, places them in organizational contexts with the particular mandate of organizational environments. These features, the institutional power structure, determine the compatibility of the ends of psychological services with the contexts in which they are implemented.

The problems of Micronesian mental health services program development addressed thus far are related to an alleged absence of psychological knowledge about the interest in the structure of behavior and the deflection of mental health personnel from duties in mental health to duties corresponding to higher-priority interests of Micronesian medical officers or interests dictated by more general sources of power including clan, island, caste, and class. These two problems, the first related to an unexamined preference for a Western institutional view of man and the second related to the necessity of implementation of development within a context of interacting traditional and bureaucratic hierarchies, are the recurrent structural problems for each of the eleven mental health services training and development programs.

PROBLEMS OF IMPLEMENTATION

An examination of the documentation of the eleven programs (grant requests, contracts, memoranda, correspondence, and one evaluation study) reveals a set of five shared characteristics across the eleven programs, as well as other programs (Robillard 1984). First, mental health services training, from 1969 to 1983, had as its primary objective the transfer of mental health services skills to Micronesian mental health coordinators or counselors or to medical officers or nurses. The recipient audience was Micronesian health care providers. The rationale for giving them these skills was based upon three interrelated assertions: that Micronesians did not possess such knowledge, that the object of professional psychology and psychiatry is the universal structure of human behavior, and that possession of this knowledge is a necessary medium for managing and intervening in human behavior, pathological and otherwise. Each successive grant request justification and training program set of objectives and methods was couched in the rhetoric of delivering services based on this reasoning.

Second, and correlatively, Micronesian cultural system versions of man and behavior had to be upgraded, and replaced with the professional scientific visions of man and behavior. Extant Micronesian cultural methods of intervention were disregarded, not even mentioned, the implicit assumption being that they are undeveloped, not yet correspondent to the empirical structure of man, that of professional psychology.

Third, as indicated in the discussion of Wilson, each successive program ran into the intricacies of the existing political economies, including the stratification systems of the various Micronesian societies. The mental health counselors were most frequently outer islanders or middle- or lower-class or -caste inner islanders. The social origin of the counselors abridged access to patients and to patient care resources, hampered the stability of the staffing of the mental health service—the counselors often being reassigned to other services by superiors—and, it was observed, decreased the likelihood that counselors would possess the psychological and cultural skills necessary to build and maintain strong mental health services offices. The trainees had no clout with hospital management, and they occupied social positions in both work and larger societal contexts that discouraged entrepreneurial assertiveness.

The social origin of the counselors was of repeated concern to the leaders of the various training programs. Notes found filed with the clinical records of the various mental health services in Micronesia indicate that some trainers perceived the low social standing of the counselors to be the cause of the failure of programs to develop in ways that had been intended (Cooper n.d.b). It was perceived by some that the wrong people had been selected and that the social mechanisms used for trainee and subsequent counselor production would continue to select the wrong individuals for mental health counseling work. It was evident that the health services were managed by higher-caste or -class individuals and that middle or lower positions were filled by individuals from ascriptively lower levels of society. The pool from which trainees would be selected would always be restricted to these middle- or lower-rank people. The higher-caste individuals who administered the health departments found it much easier to manage, in terms of rational-legal bureaucracy, lower-status individuals. Prescriptive customs of sharing of resources among higher-caste relatives are at odds with the legal constraints of Western-style management. Lower-caste individuals could not make personal claims upon the public institutions administered by members of a higher caste.

Related to the complaints of interference by the local political economies with the developmental efforts to establish mental health services is the low priority reportedly given to mental health services. The priority of mental health and the frequent reassignment of mental health personnel to other services stems from the location of power in deciding priorities. The Micronesian medical officers decide priorities, not the counselors.

Because mental health is a low priority for the M.O. managers of the health services, mental health is frequently used for other purposes. Training staff have remarked that trainees attend training programs because they provide opportunities for travel and experience. It is felt that M.O. managers hand out mental health training assignments as rewards to staff who may or may not subsequently practice in mental health services. Also, it was observed that some individuals were assigned to mental health services because they had "not worked out" in other service assignments. Mental health services were used as a vehicle to shelve incompetent people.

Significant attention was given, retrospectively or in program materials generated during implementation, to the problems of interference in program development by local social structure. If any factor can be said to have been given the blame for a failure to meet program development expectations, it is this one. However, as Dr. Anthony Polloi of Palau has cogently pointed out in reading an earlier version of this paper, no consideration had been given in retrospective program descriptions to the quality of training and development curricula and personnel. The training and development programs were not perceived by program principals as variables in the process of services development.

Fourth, an observation which is shared across the mental health training programs is that of a restricted relationship between the techniques and service modalities offered by Micronesian mental health counselors and the frequency distribution of the mental health problems experienced in Micronesia. For instance, Micronesia reportedly has the world's highest suicide rate for male adolescents and young adults (Rubinstein 1983). Training and development programs paid no attention to suicide prevention services, and there are no such services in Micronesia. The two other categories of the most frequently encountered problems are substance abuse and violence and accidents, with physical trauma often related to substance abuse. Reviews of training program curricula and allocation of training hours, as well as commentary on the outcome of the training programs, reveal but nodding attention given to these problem areas and a complete failure to establish corresponding intervention programs. Likewise, with one of the world's youngest populations, there is a complete absence of attention paid, in any of the training programs or ensuing service delivery systems, to school-related problems and the problems of children and adolescents. Curriculum design of the training programs concentrated, as stated by Wilson, in the psychopharmacological or medical interventions for psychotic behavior. The services offered, aside from not being based on an understanding or explication of local culture or language, were of a narrow spectrum, usually limited to the administration of major neuroleptic medication, e.g., prolixin. In a recent occurrence during which the hospital in the most populous state in Micronesia ran out of prolixin, mental health counselors stopped seeing patients and making home visits, explaining, "We have no medicine, there is no sense going out and wasting gas and time" (Rubinstein 1984). Mental health services in that state had become identical with the prescription of prolixin.

Fifth and finally, a common trait across the programs is that each successive program, with the exception of one, failed to mention the existence of prior efforts in mental health systems development. It is as if each effort conceptualized itself as first on the scene. Wilson and Cooper failed to mention the early training programs of 1969. McDermott failed to mention either Wilson or Summers (Gellen 1970). No one mentioned ancillary mental health services being developed in rehabilitation and special education services. Each justification for a training program, in addition to asserting a priori that professional psychological and psychiatric knowledge is essential, grounded the need for training by proclaiming Micronesians do not currently possess such knowledge. No assessments were conducted prior to training to see just what knowledge Micronesians did possess, Western or otherwise. Neither were surveys conducted to establish the dimensions of prior training and development by the navy, the Department of Interior, the Trust Territory Bureau of Health, or other vendors of services development supported by the National Institute of Mental Health.

The record of implementation reads the same across each of the training and development programs. The one exception, where a viable and stable program has evolved, is Palau. The Palau service is headed by a medical officer, not a counselor. This individual is of chiefly status in the traditional order and is joined, in the capacity of registered nurse, by a Palauan woman of the highest caste. For the rest of Micronesia, however, mental health services have suffered a 60 percent turnover in personnel. In three island groups the turnover has been over 100 percent. Moreover, as stated in state health plans and evaluations (Ponape 1983), services are restricted to the administration of neuroleptic medication and counseling, and prevention services are unavailable. Where there are clear indications of high incidence and prevalence of mental disorders related to drug and alcohol abuse, to violence and accidents, to suicide and school behavior problems, there are no services designed to meet these problems.

With this kind of track record, what explains the continuity of the programs, their repetitive or mirrorlike quality, over all the years of services development? Perhaps there is a clue to the answer to this question in the fact that each successive program operated not only unaware of structural circumstances of Micronesian cultures but also in complete ignorance of the performance of prior training programs. It is apparent that the successive training programs were loosely coupled to the social environment of Micronesia as well as to the interorganizational networks from which programs were developed, financed, and staffed (Weick 1976). What sustained this loose coupling of programs, such that programs were disjoined both from each other and from a closer articulation with the Micronesian social structures in which they were implemented? In other words, what maintains the structural balance between, on the one hand, a development advocacy of mental health services and, on the other hand, an apparent incompatibility of the implementation of such services with the circumstances of indigenous social and cultural organization?

LOOSELY JOINED NETWORKS

Perhaps the record of mental health services development in Micronesia, as well as the whole of development efforts in the area, is the consequence of being authored by those who stand at the center of American society. The people who conceived of the need to develop Micronesia, who administer the federal bureaucratic departments concerned with Micronesia (mainly the U.S. Department of Interior), those who have mastery of the institutions of the United States government and its resources, are members of what Mary Douglas and Aaron Wildavsky (1982) call the center. The constraints of such circumstances produce thought and action oriented to maintenance, at the margin, of the institutional order which is the resource base for the creation and maintenance of its members, a reflexive relationship to be found, quite naturally, within any group of similarly oriented individuals. The center is inherently conservative, and the more dense the infrastructure, the more expansive its complementary environment (Hannan and Freeman 1984) and the less probable the possibility of interaction with (no less detection of) an essentially different social order made up of an oppositional set of values at odds with the institutional order inhabited by the federal office holders, elective or administrative. The history of U.S. "development" of Micronesia, of which mental health services is but a phase, wears a very thick pair of institutional blinders, a mask so totally composed of the structural dynamics of the center that there is virtually no space and time to conceive or implement anything but the most conventional American mental health service systems.

From the assertion that development programs are the issue of those who command the complex resource base from which requisite funding is generated, it is also easy to entertain the idea that such initiatives coming from the center of the intricate capital systems which can finance such efforts are projections of the center, or core social institutions, of the society paying the bills. Those rare individuals who have expertise in the areas to be developed, those who have lived and worked in and who know the language of the developing area, are, by the time and effort taken for such a career, on the border; they are not part of the cohort whose lives have been spent mastering and elaborating the center of American administrative and financial bureaucracy. There are structural reasons why area studies specialists, anthropologists and other social scientists, and federal bureau heads, legislators, and their respective staffs fall into very different career paths (one which could be called the border and the other the center). Expertise and currency in each area is a full-time and substantively different involvement.

But is it not possible that the core or center and the border or periphery can penetrate one another? Cannot at least some of the parties to each location understand the structural dynamics in the determination of development policy and methods and correct for the problems created by invalid projections of one reality upon another?

Yes, it surely is the case that individuals from the center and the border of policy design, those who command government resources and those who are substantive experts (e.g., grass roots informants, anthropologists, and other social scientists) in the societies receiving development assistance, can come to know and utilize one another's perspectives. But we cannot merely consider the possibility of an interpenetration of such knowledge. The real question is what organizational conditions lead to such circumstances, occasions where there is mutual guidance between centrally located policymakers and those with substantive or area expertise. The type of guidance envisioned includes not only policy formulation but implementation guidance, a direction of program assembly governed by interpenetration of center and border. This kind of mutual monitoring implies a close and continuing relationship between the center and the border. Further, this kind of articulation, given the structural reasons for the separation of those in the center and the border, is rare. Each sector has its own interests and time-structured environments—respective organizational circumstances which are built, in part, by distinct mutual separation.

For instance, the assembly process of development policy formulation and implementation is both sequential and phase structured. All segments are dependent upon prior and subsequent phases, and each phase is but a step, different from but contributing to the assembly of the entire process. In the case of Micronesian development, the time, place, persons, and organizations involved in the course of investigating development needs (such as the Solomon report), debating what should be done, legislating the required funding, and recruiting administrative and line staffs for implementation for development in education, government, public works, health, or transportation are distinct sequences of action. The links between federal executive and legislative decision making, the federal agencies utilized in development, the vendors who implement the work, and those who consume and further disburse the effects of the work are, to use the phrase coined by Karl E. Weick (1976), loosely coupled. The size of the organizations and interorganizational networks involved is immense. The U.S. Department of Interior, the U.S. Congress and its subcommittees and staff, various universities, the Trust Territory of the Pacific Islands departmental staffs, and the various Micronesian state political orders are each complex, each oriented to different environments. The tight kind of relationship between center and border that would inform and monitor the conduct of development is all but impossible in the overlapping and contradictory interests and needs of all the parties involved in the development process. Additionally, each of these diverse agencies communicates with one another, and even finds the relevance in the need for mutual work by what is most general or common among them, not what is unique or esoteric to the societies of Micronesia.

Agencies interact, just as people, according to what they know of one another, guided and confirmed by acknowledgment of a mutual stock of knowledge. The repeated cycles of the projection of Western man—in terms of the psychological individual—by the entire development scheme and by, specifically, mental health services development efforts is a circumstantially limited enterprise. It is not as if psychologists and psychiatrists do not have some idea that they needed to learn more about Micronesian society before they could be truly effective. Most everyone acknowledges this need. However, programs are announced and funded with the expectation of putting in place the acknowledged services and professionals, the known architecture of mental health services. The first priority of rational action in the exchange between the funding agencies and those implementing the program is to construct the visible product which has been contracted for, the standard mental health service. Deviations from the standard, the shared expectation between all parties, would have to be worked out of ensuing interaction. The first priority is to construct and maintain common notions of professional work. Dimensions of funding and program are delimited by what is mutually known about mental health services—what is already on the shelf of shared discourse.

Further, achieving the first priority of merely getting mental health services up and running—the act before any modifications can be made—usually takes up the entire budget and exhausts the service time for each successive cohort of mental health services developers. Mental health services development is minimally funded, the amount allocated covering salaries only. Research and development are absent, as they are across the board for the creation and maintenance of health services in the Trust Territory. But even more important, the paucity of financial support and the absence of a well-developed hierarchical infrastructure of upward career mobility results in relatively short time commitments or rotations of professional mental health personnel in the Trust Territory. The development of such services is something most do as a project; the work is an activity a person moves on from after the funding elapses or a better, more stable employment comes along.

Indeed, the loosely coupled character and independent realms of needs of each of the parties involved in mental health services development (federal government legislators and administrators, program implementors, and program consumers) is exacerbated by the short-term assignment rotations of the psychiatric, psychological, and other services development providers, whether employed by the Bureau of Health Services or by university-based, grant supported projects. The cycle of turnover means that each project starts from scratch, each will tend toward the center, be a replication of the most generally accepted mental health services. The respective mental health services development staffs are passing cohorts of people for the consumers, as are the consumers for the staff. The tight integration of dependency, each cohort knowing that one possesses resources necessary for the other, does not have the chance to develop.

The misplaced concreteness indicated in the replacement of the reality of Micronesian cultural and social organization with that of professional Western psychological versions of man and experience is not a free-floating decision of mental health professionals. It is an organizationally circumscribed phenomenon. The staff funding support, the absence of adequate research and development lead time, and the supplies and support budgets of mental health services for Micronesia are limited (as they must be for any similarly situated and administered creation of a mental health service) to the first priority: the recognizable creation of professional intervention services. Any ambivalence experienced between, on the one hand, wanting to first fully analyze Micronesian cultures and, on the other hand, getting immediately on with the creation of a mental health services based on what is socially known-in-common between funding agency and implementing personnel is dissolved in the face of the limits of the dialogue between the funding agency and the professionals who are expected to set up the service. The panoply of anthropologists, linguists, sociologists, and other assorted social scientists and indigenous informants and time for extensive analysis upon which to build a mental health services program are surely not part of the mutually shared knowledge of either funding administration or professional mental health workers. What is known between them is that enough is known, though the knowledge is not complete, to set up and begin a mental health service. All parties concerned in the construction of the project know that enough is universal in their knowledge that they can and should begin.

The repeated cycling of mental health programs, limited to what is recognizable as universal to man, his structure and needs, is the outcome of interorganizational networks and mutual knowledge between those who initiate and fund services development and those who have professional knowledge in health services. To this network the cultures and societies of Micronesia are esoteric, as are those on the border of linkages between funding agencies and professional health services development, people who are on the institutional fringes of the network, like those very few who specialize in the anthropology or sociology of Micronesia. The perpetuation of the first priority of setting up a mental health service based on Western individualistic conceptions of man is a structural phenomenon, getting by on what is known among the principals of the center who initiate and carry out services development. What is not known about Micronesian cultures and languages is reserved for later, for when there might be time. But then there never is organizational time.

The centripetal force of the center, replicating the institutional structures having the greatest generality, also blinds mental health development and its parent development philosophy for Micronesia to the fact that the social history requisite to a tension between hierarchical social orders and free market or egalitarian orders (the crucible of individualism) is not present in Micronesia as it is in United States history (Wildavsky 1982). Consequently, it is difficult for a quick and successful grafting of American institutions. Micronesia is not composed of competing orders of social structure, as is true of the social history of the United States. Each of the Micronesian states remains relatively integrated along traditionally ascriptive lines. The conditions for the creation and sustenance of individuals—self-optimizing actors independent of subsumption under caste, clan, class, and ancestor attachments—are not present.

The repeated co-optation of the resources of mental health services programs by Micronesian health services management, in the form of nominating inappropriate individuals to the training programs, and the continual reassignment of mental health service personnel to other services and resulting instability of mental health services are the outcome of a web of relations between the recipient-country elite and the providers of developmental services. The high-status individuals administering the Micronesian state health services, parent bodies for mental health programs, are as much a part of the network of mutual knowledge and loose interorganizational linkages as are the professional mental health services providers/trainers and the funding agencies and superordinate congressional and executive authorities. The difference between the Micronesian health managers and those mental health professionals who contract to conduct training and development programs is that mental health is but a blip on the agenda screen of the managers, while it covers the entire screen of those who are mental health services professionals. For the Micronesian medical officer, mental health provides an insignificant amount of funding and other resources, though anything offered is accepted. While the Micronesian health bureau managers recognize that mental health services are part of the complement of health services, they also share the wider knowledge of where it fits in the priority of health services in general.

Moreover, because mental health services are an absent calculus which replaces the concrete reality of Micronesian cultural experience and because such hypostatizations are inconsequential to obtaining a better understanding, no less locating, Micronesian experience, the interpretative frame of professional mental health services has not molded itself as part and parcel of Micronesian interactional life. It is exogenous to the Micronesian experience. Mental health services are financially and programmatically, as well as in a sense of even a shared sociology of knowledge between Micronesian health administrators and funding agencies, of little importance.

CONCLUSION

With these comments in mind, is it possible to create a relevant and effective mental health service or services for the Micronesian states? We have already mentioned the influence of the center, how programs of the center are structurally limited to recreating the most general institutional structure, an organizational configuration insensitive to the unique character of Micronesian cultures and social circumstances. We have also discussed the loose network through which mental health services are implemented and consumed, how each of the main loci has its own circumstances which, in turn, limit attention and resources and make highly unlikely the possibility of the closely structured interdependencies which create mental health services within the structure of both Micronesian societies and the work of mental health services planners and implementors. We have also mentioned the dissimilarity between the social histories of the United States and Micronesia, the absence of conditions giving rise to individualism. With all these naturally occurring structural lacunae between players in the creation of mental health services, is it being overly optimistic to continue to think that services can be created and sustained at all?

Perhaps a final answer cannot be given to this question. What can be said, however, is that efforts to date have been blind, that people have been unaware of the causes and effects of programs. To even begin to speak about success in implementing a mental health service system, a theory of organization and interorganizational systems must be articulated; a theory of how to create linkages which insure an increasingly complex system of reciprocal experience encompassing both Western mental health constructs and Micronesian phenomenology. To date, the evidence is that mental health services efforts have proceeded with the naivete of the expansion of the center, an expansion resulting in more than mere ethnocentrism—resulting, instead, in rational but superficial development among a network of organizational actors, never becoming a piece of Micronesian operational culture and social structure.

APPENDIX: MENTAL HEALTH DEVELOPMENT PROGRAMS

1969, Mental Health Training Program for Micronesian Health Services. Dr. Torres Hospital, Saipan, Northern Marianas. Training in general principles of mental health counseling. Trainees included policemen, Head Start personnel, village commissioners, and mental health counselors. Dr. Gerhardt Summers, director of Division of Mental Health, Trust Territory of the Pacific Islands Bureau of Health Services, led the program. The program was seven weeks in duration (Gellen 1970).

1974–1978, Micronesian Mental Health Coordinators Training Program. Six Micronesian paraprofessional health workers, mostly practical nurses and health aides, were selected and trained in basic principles of psychology and medical management of psychiatric problems by Dr. Larry Wilson and R. CeCilia Cooper, both of the Division of Mental Health. The training consisted of "twelve to eighteen hours of initial instruction" followed by regular visits by the supervising psychiatrist and psychologist, where practicum instruction would take place over five days, and an occasional workshop to address counseling techniques. Psychopharmacological management was the focal point of training (Wilson 1981).

1977–1979, Mental Health Training Program, Bureau of Health Services, Trust Territory of the Pacific Islands. Financed by a grant of $96,096 from the United States National Institute of Mental Health, the program offered three levels of education: (1) existing mental health staffs in Micronesia; (2) community influentials; and (3) the public at large. Trainees from within the departments of Health, Education, Public Safety, and Community Development, as well as the clergy, were trained in basic concepts of mental health, communications skills, crisis intervention, and in mass media techniques for educating the general public to deal with stress and other conflicts (NIMH 1984). Mental health coordinators were sent to Seattle Central Community College for a year and then on to Stanford University for training in mass communication techniques. Coordinators from Yap, the Marshalls, and Saipan were enrolled (de Brum 1984).

1978–1981, Cross-Cultural Counseling Training, Institute of Behavioral Sciences, Honolulu, Hawaii. Supported by a grant of $320,540 from the U.S. National Institute of Mental Health, a private, not-for-profit research organization composed largely of University of Hawaii faculty offered training in cross-cultural counseling. The National Institute of Mental Health memo reporting this program states, "there was a good representation of trainees from other Pacific Basic jurisdictions" (1984). Inquiries to the principals of this training program reveal an absence of Pacific Islander participants from jurisdictions beyond Hawaii. The program is listed here, nevertheless, because it expressed the superficial development of mental health services for the Trust Territories, the overly expansive representation about mental health services development for Pacific Islanders when in fact no such development had taken place.

1979, Prototype Psychiatric Training for Medical Officers. A contract training program conducted by the University of Hawaii Department of Psychiatry for the Trust Territory of the Pacific Islands was designed to train two Micronesian medical officers for six months of psychiatry (McDermott 1979).

1980–1983, Psychiatric Training for Trust Territory Medical Officers. With an award of $176,318 from the U.S. National Institute of Mental Health, the University of Hawaii Department of Psychiatry expanded short-term residency-level training of Micronesian medical officers (McDermott 1979). The program was designed to train fourteen additional medical officers. At completion of the program, five individuals had matriculated.

1980–1981, Forensic Training for Pacific Basin Jurisdictions. Financed by a $17,000 supplement to a Center for Manpower Development, NIMH, grant awarded to the State of Hawaii, medical officers and nurses from the Marshall Islands, Palau, and Guam were brought to Honolulu to attend a week-long conference in forensic psychiatry (NIMH 1984).

1979–1980, Loma Linda University Mental Health Services and Training. The Department of Psychiatry of Loma Linda University School of Medicine established a psychiatric residency rotation in tropical psychiatry. The site for the training was at MacDonald Memorial Hospital in Koror, Palau. One resident completed the rotation (Kaunders 1980a, 1980b). The objectives of expanding the scope and number of trainees in the rotation have not materialized.

1982, Mental Health Counselor Training Workshop, Ponape. Supported by Trust Territory of the Pacific Islands Bureau of Health Services funding of $7,711, three University of Hawaii Department of Psychiatry faculty conducted a week long workshop in mental health counseling to four Micronesian mental health counselors/coordinators.

1982–1983, Pacific Island Mental Health Counselor Training Program. With an award from the National Institute of Mental Health for a grant of

$59,960, twelve mental health counselors from the Trust Territory of the Pacific Islands and American Samoa were brought to Honolulu for nine weeks of training. The training was conducted by the University of Hawaii Department of Psychiatry (Robillard 1984). An evaluation of services outcome of the training was conducted during the summer of 1983.

1982–1983, Pacific Islander Alternative Mental Health Services. With the objective of designing and evaluating alternative mental health services, a grant of $60,000 was awarded by the National Institute of Mental Health to the University of Hawaii Department of Psychiatry to work with the mental health services of the Micronesian state health departments.

Two other components of mental health services development should be mentioned. First, national institutes of Mental Health, Alcohol Abuse and Alcoholism, and Drug Abuse funding provided $587,000 for services for the Trust Territory for the 1972–1983 period (NIMH 1984). This amount is in addition to the project grants listed above. The funding was granted by manpower development and clinical treatment programs within the three institutes. While the total amount of funding may not seem large, it must be understood in the context of being spread over 125,000 people and in economies, such as in Truk, where the starting minimum wage in 1983 was but seventy-five cents per hour and the average yearly per capita income substantially below one thousand dollars.

Second, there occurred during the same time frame, 1969–1983, other training and development programs which had a direct relationship to creating mental health services capacity. The University of Guam Division of Nursing, for example, in 1982 conducted a training program in psychiatric nursing for Palau. The course was designed to enhance the ability of Palauan nurses to pass mental health and psychiatric content portions of the United States national licensure board examinations for licensed practical nurses (LPN). Another training program with mental health services components was a vocational rehabilitation counselor program. Counselors from each island district have been recruited and trained in Honolulu, in the Marshall Islands, and in Guam. An ostensible goal of vocational rehabilitation counseling is to serve the chronically mentally ill.

Translating Primary Health Care Policies to the Local Level: A Comparison of Rural Communities in the United States and Costa Rica

Carole E. Hill

Primary Health Care (PHC) has been hailed as the answer to most of the world's health problems.[1] The Alma-Ata International Conference on PHC held in Moscow in 1978 defined it as essential health care with at least eight components.[2] This new health initiative would draw sustenance from four principal strategies: (1) political commitment, (2) community participation, (3) concerted action among various sectors of development, and (4) appropriate choice of technology. By recognizing that health is more than a medical issue, the PHC initiative broadens the traditional medical model of delivering health care. It means nutrition, sanitation, clean water, maternal and child care, contraceptives and family planning, immunizations, education, and appropriate technology. It is health care that is accessible, acceptable, and affordable with an emphasis on promotive and preventive services while delivering curative and rehabilitative services. PHC, ideally, is the first contact point between the patient and the health system. It is more than delivering health as a product to the people. Instead, it looks at health in its social and cultural setting and in the context of issues much wider than those which the health services have conventionally tried to tackle (WHO and UNICEF 1978).

If the PHC model of health care is to be translated to the community level, changes in the traditional medical model as well as changes in the patterns of resource allocation have to take place. Indeed, "it is because the existing pattern of resource allocation in the health care sector reflects real and not imagined interests, that altering this pattern by political means is the litmus test of national commitment to PHC" (WHO and UNICEF 1978). In this paper I will compare the PHC policies in rural areas for two countries—the United States and Costa Rica—and evaluate how they have been translated to the community level. The policy process involves finding solutions to public health problems (the solution to a specific problem is chosen from a variety of alternatives), implementing the solution (programs), and evaluating the results. This paper will analyze and compare the implementation and evaluative phases of this process and make some suggestions for alternative policies for more efficient implementation (translation) of PHC on the community level. First, however, I will briefly discuss the PHC policies in Costa Rica and the United States. Data were collected in a rural community in Georgia (for the sake of anonymity called "Coberly") and two rural communities in Costa Rica (El Puente and Caribe).

PRIMARY HEALTH CARE POLICIES IN RURAL AREAS: UNITED STATES AND COSTA RICA

In Costa Rica, health care, social security, and free primary school education are considered the "pillars of the democratic system." Therefore, the state developed a highly centralized and coordinated health system with a wide coverage of the population during the 1970s as a response to a growing popular demand for health services. They accomplished this without jeopardizing the basic promises of a capitalist structure. Within a basic capitalistic economic system, the health system of Costa Rica is very close to being a national health service (table 1). It has two structures that deliver health service—the Social Security System and the Ministry of Health. In 1961, a constitutional amendment was passed calling for social security to reach universal coverage in ten years. Between 1962 and 1966 coverage was given to most rural areas, and in the 1970s the system expanded in order to create the administrative and legal structure necessary for the integration of medical care under social security for the entire population.

Table 1

Health Sector: Institutions According to Dependency and Category, 1979

Type of Institution	Dependency	Number
National hospitals—general	Social Security System	4
National hospitals—specialized	Social Security System	5
Regional hospitals	Social Security System	9
Regional hospitals	Ministry of Health	1
Area hospitals	Social Security System	7
Periphery hospitals	Social Security System	2
Out-patient clinics	Social Security System	84
Health centers	Ministry of Health	78
Health centers—Rural Assistance	Ministry of Health	4
Nutritional and education centers (CEN)	Ministry of Health	501
Integral infants center of attention (CINAI)	Ministry of Health	34
Educational and nutritional recuperation centers (CERN)	Ministry of Health	1
Nutritional recuperation clinics	Ministry of Health (INCIENSA)	1
Rural health posts	Ministry of Health	287
Rural health posts	Ministry of Health (San Ramon Prog.)	45
Rural health posts	Social Security System	3
Outpatient clinics for alcoholics	Ministry of Health (INSA)	1
Alcoholic rehabilitation center	Ministry of Health (INSA)	1
Dental clinics—(directed to schools)	Ministry of Health	29
Dental clinics—health centers	Ministry of Health	32
Odontology mobile units	Ministry of Health	43
Medical mobile units	Ministry of Health	12
Private clinics	Private	3

Source: Memoria 1979, Ministry of Health

Although the system (created in 1941) had extended medical services to people in the national and provincial capitals who earned less than four hundred colones a month, service to rural workers was gradually extended outside the central valley (by 1961, 18 percent of the total population had sickness and maternal coverage). The system subsequently built its own hospitals and outpatient services (mostly in the San Jose area) and retained salaried physicians and health workers (often buying services from charity hospitals). In the 1970s it took over all the charity hospitals in the provincial areas and San Jose and the banana company hospitals in the lowland areas. By 1975, over 90 percent of the country's doctors were employees of the Social Security System (about one-third have some sort of private practice). All salaried workers and others who opted to join the system are required to pay a monthly charge. Other forms of finance besides employee quotas include revenues from the lottery and increased governmental subsidies.

The Ministry of Health (MH) is responsible for all primary care given under the community and rural health program initiated in 1973. Health posts were established in communities with populations less than one thousand and number 287 for the country. The staff consists of a traveling physician, an auxiliary nurse, and a health assistant whose duties are to keep house-by-house records of families in the area, provide health education, keep track of immunizations, and refer acute and chronically ill patients to social security (CCSS) clinics and hospitals. In addition, the MH is responsible for sanitary programs such as insect control, malaria, food and drug control, environmental programs, child nutrition, and VD. The MH administers only 20 percent of the total national expenditure in health. With these funds, it is to serve 20 percent of the urban population and 30 percent of the rural population not presently covered by the Social Security System. (It also serves many people who are insured. In 1978, 770,000 rural dwellers were visited or treated by rural health assistants.) The health posts give outpatient care such as prenatal and well-child consultation, family planning, basic dental care, and immunization and directly carry out control programs for special diseases such as tuberculosis and malaria. They are considered the "gateway" into the health care system (figure 1). These allocations of duties between the two systems were made with the understanding that the long-term goal would be the cre-

Figure 1
Levels of Attention

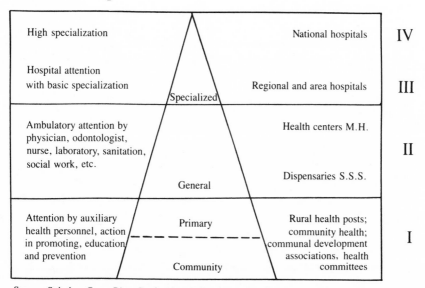

High specialization		National hospitals	IV
Hospital attention with basic specialization	Specialized	Regional and area hospitals	III
Ambulatory attention by physician, odontologist, nurse, laboratory, sanitation, social work, etc.	General	Health centers M.H. / Dispensaries S.S.S.	II
Attention by auxiliary health personnel, action in promoting, education and prevention	Primary / Community	Rural health posts; community health; communal development associations, health committees	I

Source: *Salud en Costa Rica: Evaluacion de la situacion en la decada de los años 70.* Ministerio de Salud Unidad de Planificacion, 1981, San Jose, Costa Rica.

ation of one integrated health system. The two systems are now coordinated by a National Health Council (Casas and Vargas 1980).

Although the office of the Secretary of Health, Education, and Welfare offered us a Forward Plan for Health Report in 1974 that included a goal of preparing for a national health system, the U.S. system is decentralized and pluralistic and is neither centrally structured (except for federal and state programs that are legally defined by federal and state regulations) nor centrally financed. It includes both public and private financing and almost every conceivable kind of organizational arrangement. There is no general health law which specifies health care that is to be provided at the state or local level (Berg et al. 1976), although the idea that health care is a right and not a privilege was a strong basis for much of the legislation in the 1960s and 1970s. In the United States, the various bodies concerned with organization, financing, and evaluation of health care delivery have only very tentative lines of authority and communication, although there is a considerable amount of informal coordination. "However, the health care situation in the U.S. is disputed and coordinated. There is no single pool of health care monies and no central authority to negotiate its expenditures" (Berg et al. 1976).

Unlike Costa Rica, the democratic government of the United States has yet to discover how to develop such a system without feeling it would jeopardize the principle of capitalism. Consequently, most health services are provided on the basis of fee-for-service or co-payments through insurance or HMO. A majority of physicians are in private practice and have the power to charge what they want for services. Only the poor and elderly qualify for Medicaid or Medicare, programs enacted at the national level of government to provide health care for the underprivileged. These programs, administered through national and state agencies, increased the access to health care of a segment of the population but did not restructure the general health care system (but did begin the economic restructuring based on corporate financing for profit making). In addition to these private services, some services are administered through federal regulations, others through state structures and regulations.

Until the 1970s, the PHC existent in rural areas had been delivered through the Public Health System. In the rural South, sanitation programs were carried out in the early 1900s that screened for insects and protected water supplies (decreasing incidence of typhoid fever), a part of the Rural Sanitation Act of 1916. In the following decades, public health services focused their efforts in nuclear waste control and community sanitation. The medical personnel were employed by the Public Health Service, which began to attack what it deemed the major problem facing rural families—the lack of adequate medical services—by developing programs of rural rehabilitation which they felt would improve the poor economic conditions of many rural areas (Williams 1951).

In the 1950s public health efforts began to focus on increasing institutional services to rural populations and away from communicable diseases (for example, the Hospital Survey and Construction Act of 1950). For two decades, the policy emphasis in rural areas focused on secondary care with most of the PHC administered by a public health nurse in the state-regulated clinic or a private doctor. In the 1970s, Rural Health Initiative Programs were passed and administered by the Public Health Service. The purpose of the programs is to develop and systematize the delivery of health care in rural areas. The programs included under this act are (1) National Health Service Corporation, (2) Migrant Health Program, (3) Community Health Centers, (4) Health for Underserved Rural Areas Program, and (5) Appalachian Health Programs. Small clinics have been constructed with national funds and staffed generally by physicians paid by the National Health Service Corporation. The programs were paid for by using tax monies, a kind of redistributing income for equity in access and availability.

To coordinate health planning and resource development in regions within states, Congress passed The National Health Planning and Resources Development Act of 1974, establishing Health System Agencies (HSA) which were required to develop a Health System Plan and Annual Implementation Plan (AIP) for the region. Although HSAs are in the process or have "gone out of business," community groups who requested funds for PHC clinics had to go through these agencies. Indeed, the community I studied in rural Georgia qualified as an Underserved Rural Area and the funds for a PHC were funneled through the HSA in the region. It should be noted that some of these programs are no longer operational and funding has been severely cut.

The services ideally provided by the PHC, as stated in the proposal for the establishment of a clinic in Coberly, include (1) family planning, (2) well-adult care with the main objectives being preventive, early detection and patient education, and to establish linkages with health advocacy agencies, (3) services for disease known to be prevalent in the population, (4) well-child care focusing on prevention of childhood disease through immunization, (5) prenatal care to pregnant women, (6) chronic disease care, (7) hypertension treatment, (8) preventive dental care, (9) emergency medical services, (1) nutritional programs, (11) health education, (12) transportation, (13) social services to be used as linkages to other agencies, (14) supplemental laboratory services, (15) specialty medical consultation in adjacent counties, (16) hospital service in adjacent counties, (17) pharmacy services, (18) home health care, (19) extended care facilities, and (20) evaluation procedures. Not all these services are provided in the community of Coberly, as I will discuss later. The services that are provided are paid for on a fee-for-service basis with a sliding scale or through Medicare and Medicaid. The goal of these clinics is to become economically self-sufficient within a three-year period.

HEALTH PROBLEMS AND HEALTH STATUS IN
THE COMMUNITIES

The most important variables that affect health status, particularly in developing nations, are distribution of wealth, level of education, sanitation, housing conditions, life-style (Elling 1978) and access to health facilities. Indeed, health status is more an indicator than a symptom of inequality. Rural areas generally share a common predicament—they are underserved and the quality of health care is inferior to that found in urban access (Carballo 1978). Most of the health problems in the communities in Costa Rica and the United States are either chronic or environmental; problems that are treatable by services supposedly provided for under the concept of PHC. The majority are community based rather than biologically based.

The communities in Costa Rica are located in one of the most underdeveloped areas of the country, and the community in the United States is located in the traditional plantation area of the old South. All communities have a high unemployment rate (circa 10 percent). In 1980, Coberly's median household income was $6,652 with 27 percent below the poverty level, and the median income in Costa Rica was $1,732 and under $500 in the communities of Caribe and El Puente. Although income is relative to a specific country, all the communities studied are poor when compared to the median income in the respective nations.

The mortality rates in Coberly indicate that the leading causes of death are heart disease, cancer, and cerebrovascular disease. In Caribe and El Puente the major causes of death are heart disease and cerebrovascular and respiratory problems for adults and infections in the postnatal period for infants. Furthermore, the major health problems in all communities are high blood pressure, diabetes, obesity, and mental stress, with parasites being a major problem in Caribe and El Puente. Other statistics reveal that in the U.S. community, socioeconomic and ethnic status are directly related to health. For example, in 1980 "Cober County" had an infant mortality of 70 deaths per 1,000 for blacks and 0 for whites, while the rate for neonatal deaths was 46.5 per 1,000 for blacks and 12.1 per 1,000 for whites. The infant mortality rate in Costa Rica has improved drastically over the past ten years (from 61.5 per 1,000 in 1970 to 18.3 in 1983), and it has improved within all regions in the Limon Province (Caribe and El Puente) except the one in which Caribe is located (the community furthest away from Puerto Limon). The rate here was 56.4 per 1,000 (statistics are not broken up into ethnic categories). The infant mortality rates, however, are currently on the rise. Early in 1984, infant mortality had risen to 18.2 per 1,000, which the minister of health feels is due to the economic crisis (Mesoamerica 1984).

Casas and Vargas (1980) state that 20 percent of the population have no access to elementary health services in Costa Rica. The life expectancy for both countries is almost the same—73.2 for Costa Rica and 74.5 for the United States (Jaramillo 1983). Sanitation is a major problem in the Costa Rican communities and not so much a problem in the United States, while housing is a problem in the United States communities (40 percent of houses are considered to be overcrowded) and not a major problem in the Costa Rican communities, except among the very poor. Finally, a large percentage of the people are not covered by any form of health insurance—25 percent for El Puente and Caribe and 20 percent for Coberly. A survey by the Census Bureau found only 51 percent of nonmetropolitan households reported any member with health insurance coverage and 39 percent reported a member with a pension plan (Current Population Reports 1982). Lastly, the county in which Coberly is located had been without the services of a doctor for fifteen years before the PHC clinic hired one in 1982.

TRANSLATING POLICIES TO THE LOCAL LEVEL

The implementation of the PHC policies on the local level has proven to be difficult in both countries for a variety of reasons, the major problems being economic and organizational. I conducted research in rural communities in the United States and Costa Rica to discover the problems of the PHC system and will report the major problems I discovered in the system as well as the people's perspective on problems with the system.

Costa Rica

It is impossible to fully understand the dynamics of the health care system in Costa Rica without linking it with international monetary policies. For example, the country recently signed an agreement with the International Monetary Fund pledging the state to reduce all its expenditures, particularly health, education, and social welfare programs. But for the purpose of this paper, I will only discuss the national and regional levels. In 1970, 3 percent of the gross national product was spent on health; in 1979, the percentage rose to 6 percent. In 1977, the social security budget was 63 percent of the country's total health expenditures, and the MH received less than one-fourth of the total sum. Indeed, in the last ten years the MH budget has doubled while the social security expeditures rose 560 percent (Casas and Vargas 1980). In 1980, the MH budget was cut by 10 percent, a comment on the priorities the state places on secondary and tertiary care as opposed to PHC, although the policies have always been oriented toward curative services. Indeed, four times more resources are now allocated to hospital and ambulatory care than for preventive medicine. Within this framework, however, the Rural Health Program has done much more to lower infant mortality and malnutrition than the social security clinics and regional hospitals (Casas and Vargas 1980:276).

Another major problem involves the organization, or lack of it. The people of Caribe simply cannot depend on the health post to systematically service their health problems. The regional physician had no transportation for months. He would borrow the dentist's jeep for unscheduled visits to health posts in the area. The physician's territory ranged from the Nicaraguan border in the north to near the Panamanian border to the south. So, unless the people had money for transportation and participated in the social security system, they rarely, if ever, had access to health services. Scheduling is also a problem. For example, the health post in El Puente was scheduled to have fifteen visits by the mobile medical unit in 1983, and during the first eight months of the year, it was open only six days. The health post in Caribe (located at least an hour's ride from Puerto Limon) was utilized more by the local population than the one in El Puente, located about twenty-five minutes away from Puerto Limon.

During three months in 1983, the health field study post in Caribe was open for a week at one time with the doctor present. A total of fifty-seven people saw him during this time. The nurse often opened the health post for consultation, when the doctor was not present. She consulted sometimes up to forty persons per day. Other times, the doctor was available, infrequently. In El Puente, the health post opened daily for the nutritional program, and the health assistant often consulted with the mothers and with others who would walk or ride the train from outlying areas. We observed people coming from outlying areas daily only to find the health post closed. Furthermore, we found that the people in the outlying areas attempted to use the health post more frequently than the ones who lived in the communities (the closer they lived, the less likely to use the health posts). Children and women between the ages of twenty and forty-four used it much more frequently than older women or men of all ages (mostly due to the nutritional program), and whites used it more frequently than blacks. They often walked miles to the health post only to find it closed.

The field study in 1984 revealed very little change in the utilization patterns but a few substantial changes in the personnel and delivery of care. The new doctor, originally from the community, has taken an extraordinary interest in the health of the people. She has transportation and attempts to maintain the schedule posted on the doors of the health posts in her territory. She has activated the health committee and an auxiliary worker has been hired. Such enthusiasm is tempered, however, by the sparsity of medicine and equipment.

In addition to transportation and overextension of the personnel, other problems exist with the health posts. The one in Caribe did not have a health assistant or an auxiliary worker for over a year. Consequently, the records were not up-to-date and no one reached out to the communities. In addition, medicines are low in supply, some do not exist, and all are relatively old; very little equipment can be found in the health posts. Furthermore, the physicians frequently refer their patients to the clinic in Puerto Limon, mostly because they are usually young and inexperienced with rural health problems. The people are aware of these referral patterns and feel that they can save time and money if they go directly to the hospital or clinic in Puerto Limon first.

Consequently, the people of Caribe have little or no primary health care and absolutely no health promotion services. They perceive the PHC system to be unreliable and undependable and have a general lack of confidence in it. As previously stated, according to the health care providers and the records in the health posts, the major health problems in the communities are high blood pressure, parasites, malnutrition, arthritis, low blood pressure, and stress, all of which require primary health care and health promotion. Other health problems in the communities are the result of sanitary conditions and the living conditions of the very poor (overcrowding, no shoes, poorly designed latrines, etc.), situations that cannot be changed by the PHC system as it currently is organized.

The people's perspective about the solution to these problems with the health care system demonstrates to me at least that they have some understanding of the health problems. The most frequently suggested change in the system is to have a permanent physician in the communities; this is followed by the suggestion to have a permanent nurse and more medicines at the health posts. Furthermore, they suggested better equipment and more reliable schedules for the health post. All these suggestions involve the health post, the most underutilized health resource in the community. The remaining suggestions involve the community level and the overall health delivery system and include health education in schools; more interest and participation by a community health committee, especially in regard to environmental health conditions in the community (better water and sanitary system); and general improvement of living conditions, especially economic conditions.

United States

Unlike Costa Rica, the health system in the United States, a developed nation, does not depend on the International Monetary Fund and, as a consequence, is dependent on its own policies and ideally is accountable only to its population. In 1982, health costs reached $322 million, or about 10.5% of the GNP, a cost that is viewed as having gotten out of hand. Measures are being taken by the government to curtail this growth by restructuring the reimbursement regulations to hospitals. Instead of reimbursing hospitals for the costs of treating each patient, the state will pay a fixed but different amount for each type of medical problem, regardless of how much service the patient actually receives. Although this change will revolutionize the economics of hospital care, it only affects the secondary and tertiary levels of medicine. Efforts to curtail the cost of private medical care are, at the present time, mostly ideological—ranging from suggested policies to regulate or freeze the charges of physicians and private hospitals and clinics to a laissez-faire policy that believes in the equity of the market.

For example, the priority research areas for health services research in fiscal year 1984 will "continue to include evaluation of strategies to encourage healthful behavior, the role of competition and productivity in the health market place and improvement in health delivery methods" (HSR Reports 1983:4).

The recent economic policies have impacted the PHC in rural areas. First, the HSAs have been dismantled, and the states have been given the responsibility to support, structure, and plan for primary health care in rural areas. The state of Georgia does not have a separate department for rural health service as opposed to urban health service; thus, rural areas are planned for by each of the six sections in the Division of Public Health. The section most responsible for developing and coordinating the policies is, of course, the Primary Health Care Section. It now finds itself having to play a greater role in the financing of the PHC clinics that were originally financed by the national government. Consequently, similar to organizational problems in Costa Rica, the state is now helping to support two clinics in Coberly that virtually compete with one another for patients. One, the Public Health Clinic, traditionally funded by the state level of government, offers limited services at a minimal or no charge. The PHC clinic, on the other hand, has problems offering services that would be considered basic PHC services. For the most part it offers mostly curative medicine, and although the extreme organizational problems discovered in Caribe and El Puente do not exist in Coberly and the majority of people had access to medical care, they are still at a higher risk for health problems than those in urban areas, and they are, in actuality, receiving only selected PHC services.

Most people in the town depend upon Medicare or Medicaid for the payment of health services if they utilize the PHC clinic, and the remaining people use private physicians. There are a significant number of people who could not afford a comprehensive health plan and do not qualify for entitlement programs. (Nineteen percent of the population reportedly use Medicaid/Medicare, 31 percent are considered indigent, and 50 percent use private insurance; in addition, 50 percent of the population made under $10,000 in 1980.) If they had coverage at all, it was for hospitalization. The very poor, mostly women who seek family planning or prenatal/postnatal care, continue to use the Public Health Clinic. Both men and women utilize the Public Health Clinic for blood pressure checkups, and children are taken to clinic for immunizations.

Because these two clinics are in competition for patients and some patients "shop around" both within and outside the county, complete health records are not available for patients. According to the health workers, this is the major problem of organization in the community. Before this occurred, however, there were problems in finding a physician for PHC clinics (it took over a year to secure one), and, after the physician arrived, the nurse practitioner who had attended to patients for a year left and was not replaced (the director said, "Now that we have a doctor, he can take care of the clientele"). The physician had difficulty obtaining hospital privileges in the nearby facility.

Furthermore, because of the regulation that the clinic will have twenty-four-hour coverage and cannot use the hospital for backup, the physician is literally on duty twenty-four hours. Indeed, the director of the clinic was told by the doctors in nearby hospitals that they did not support the idea of a PHC facility and resented the use of taxpayers' monies to build a clinic they felt was not needed. As a consequence of these organizational problems, it has been difficult to establish linkages to other parts of the health system. The health promotions and screening activities were dropped due to the lack of a nurse practitioner, making the PHC clinic basically a curative one with little or no outreach into the community. As in Costa Rica, the extensive services supposedly offered by the PHC clinic were cut to treating outpatients—services which were paid for through entitlement programs.

Most of the people of Coberly have continued to use their own physicians (outside the county), and many (20 percent) do not feel that there was a need for the PHC clinic. As in any rural community, they are surprised at these "outsiders" who try to change things, and the people who are considered the "outsiders" do not tend to hire local people ("No qualified person could be found to employ within the county," according to the director). The locals feel that the few people who worked to bring the clinic to the community did so for their own personal gain. I surveyed the community months after the clinic had opened. Forty percent were not aware of its existence, and 25 percent said that they would not use the clinic except in emergency cases. Most felt that the PHC clinic would be a "welfare clinic."

A large number of people use emergency rooms in nearby hospitals for PHC needs which, in addition to the use of private doctors, indicates that most people are "getting into the health care system at the wrong end." Although the program of maternal and infant care is ostensibly a viable program in all the Public Health Clinics in the state, actual delivery under the Medicaid program is done only in five hospitals. Therefore, the people have to travel long distances for delivery. Most do not. Therefore, they receive minimal, if any, prenatal services and generally just show up at the nearest emergency room. Like the people of El Puente and Caribe in Costa Rica, the people of Coberly base their decision about the services they use for health problems on their experience and knowledge, perceptions and evaluation of good health care, perceived seriousness of illness, cost and method of payment, and accessibility. They do not use the rational model of health-seeking behavior the planners had in mind when they felt that the entrance into the system would be through the primary level.

IMPLEMENTING POLICY AND PROGRAM ALTERNATIVES

Must I say the obvious? In order to improve the health status of people in rural areas, especially the poor, changes must occur on both the macro- and microlevels of policy construction and implementation in the communities. Since they are dependent on the policies of the larger systems, I suggest that the impetus for change must come from the state in terms of resource allocation and enforcement of PHC policies. The major problems in both countries stem from a hegemonic domination of an urban-based, economically privileged class, which includes the medical system, and the ideology that legitimizes its power. Because this system is so entrenched in the beliefs of the policymakers, the ideology and practices are very difficult to alter (Gramsci 1971).

Policies and programs originating in the urban area can, according to Malloy and Borzutsky (1982), create increased social stratification. They feel that in Latin American countries, the rural areas have not been adequately covered by the social security system—health facilities are often concentrated in urban areas with a bias toward curative medicine, and thus only a limited sector of the population has access to the health system. They refer to this phenemenon as the "hierarchical pattern of coverage among the insured" (1982:93). I found this process to exist not only in Costa Rica but also in the rural areas of the United States.

Health care policies are constructed and their enforcement, consequently, depends to a large extent on the cultural system of the policy makers (who, in Costa Rica, historically ignored the Limon area). The beliefs and practices of the dominant classes in the communities are much more congruent with the ideology of the external system than are those of the lower-class groups. In implementing a PHC model and thus expanding the dominant medical system (which increases the expectations of the people), the principles of community-based organization, use of local health workers, and traditional medicines must be implemented. Otherwise, such intervention runs the risk of shifting the people's awareness away from the nonmedical causes of illness and disease to a medical explanation (the biomedical ideology). Furthermore, it runs a high risk of being ineffectual. As stated earlier, the people in the communities are quite capable of evaluating and judging the PHC system. The content of the health promotion and education component must be operationalized in a feasible and appropriate manner. Although the beliefs and practices of the people in the communities incorporate the dominant model, they are not limited by it. Such beliefs and practices (including indigenous technology) are resources for developing a PHC program.

Furthermore, most people in the communities want equal opportunities and participation in the structuring of their health world. And although increasing access and expanding community programs expands the culture and structure of the dominant system, such programs link people with divergent health beliefs and practices and allow for the beginning of alternative pathways to health. Perhaps this is one of the main reasons for not implementing the key concepts of PHC. It would mean that in the translation process various ideologies would be negotiated—a give-and-take of the various cultural and social systems legitimizing their interdependence and mutual contributions toward improving health.

It should be kept in mind that a community is rarely homogeneous; there are varying levels of socioeconomic groups in communities, and since the basic instrumental mechanism for access and participation in the health system is economic status, there will be people who have access and others who do not. Therefore, a model of community participation must include all groups, not just the leaders who in the United States are often satisfied with the health care delivery system. Lack of support and organization for PHC in rural areas appears to be a political and economic question, not a medical one. It means (1) bringing the poor into the planning and decision-making process, (2) increased allocation of funds, and (3) changes in health ideology. In discussing community participation for health, De Kadt (1984) concludes that for Latin America, at least, participation will only thrive under governments with a strong commitment to overcoming poverty and social inequality. Often, "the poor are made to share the burden of providing for their own health need, while there is little or no change in the biased allocation of government resources to hospitals and (urban) curative care" (De Kadt 1984:244).

These suggestions for implementing PHC programs are aimed at the national policy level. They include a kind of health praxis in which the links between the health circumstances of rural people and the actions needed to change these circumstances can be realized. Such an approach is grounded in the ability of the people to reflect upon their health conditions and to take actions for change if given the opportunity and freedom to do so. Rational health praxis, based on a systems theory of social order and change, would involve people on all levels of the health hierarchy and, importantly, would take the social and cultural system of the people—both the policymakers and the community people—into consideration. I argue that the PHC system needs to be transformed for the purpose of (1) increasing equity: (2) increasing individual, family, and community health knowledge and wellness; (3) continually protecting and promoting health; (4) organizing health care services and technology appropriate for the community/regional level; and (5) integrating people and health institutions.

For the United States' health system, I suggest the following policy and program alternatives:

1. Health structure/services. These changes include (a) the training and utilization of rural health teams (including local traditional healers), (b) participation of community people from all segments of the social structure and of health planners and policymakers, (c) efficient management (multi-task oriented), (d)

linking mental health and physical health services, and (e) changing criteria for underserved areas to a regional level rather than the county level.

2. Health personnel. These changes include (a) restructuring PHC teams to include medical and nonmedical personnel (i.e., nurse practitioners, psychiatric social workers, dentists, nutritionists, pharmacists, community paraprofessionals, community life-style advisors, ministers, and representatives from community/regional organizations), (b) personnel trained in preventive health techniques which include indigenous ones, (c) selection of teams based on epidemiological surveys of the key health problems of the community and on sociocultural studies about knowledge, attitudes, expectations, beliefs, and behavior about health, (d) existing paraprofessionals and community representatives given incentives to participate in health teams, and (e) increased incentives for doctors, nurses, and dentists to locate in rural areas (on federal and state levels).

3. Cost structure. These changes include (a) implementation of a national health insurance that entitles all citizens to comprehensive health care, (b) public and private insurance plans to develop and fund efforts to establish HMO-type systems in rural areas, (c) elimination of the differences between rural and urban reimbursement rates to doctors and nurse practitioners in Medicare and Medicaid programs, (d) change in eligibility requirements for medical aid to rural areas to better fit the cultural and social situation (i.e., development of policies that will ensure that medical personnel can be reimbursed for the PHC services) and that are linked to secondary and tertiary levels of health, and (e) provision of incentives for overall economic development including adequate housing and ecological and sanitation standards.

4. Technical structure. These changes include (a) development of a research center and clearinghouse in different regions of the state to conduct research and monitor and evaluate health programs, (b) provision for periodic conferences, seminars, and short courses for jointly organized representatives from all levels of the PHC system, and (c) establishment of telecommunications with regional hospitals and other secondary and tertiary care units.

The policy and program alternatives I suggest for Costa Rica are not as extensive as for the United States, since its existing policies ideally support a rather unified approach to PHC. Indeed, Caribe has a health committee that attempts to become involved in the health problems of the community but is encouraged only to raise funds for cleaning and buying equipment for the health post. This involvement is only superficial. Therefore, I recommend that the existing policies be implemented with the following recommendations:

1. Decrease the territory covered by the physician in a region, and increase the number of physicians.
2. Increase the supply of medicines in the health post, and rotate medicines that are not dispensed within a certain time frame.
3. Provide reliable transportation for the physician, nurse, and dentist.
4. Extend mental health services to the rural areas.
5. Implement a preventive health program that considers the cultural and environmental context of the communities for children and adults (not just low-weight infants or pregnant women).
6. Involve community groups and individuals in the planning and implementation of health care, including representatives from all segments of the community.
7. Strengthen the health committees in the communities through projects such as waste disposal and clean water.
8. Integrate the use of natural plants and natural healers into a unified approach.

SUMMARY

Both governments (United States and Costa Rica) continue to support a two-class system of medicine and appear to be heading toward maintaining such a system. Particularly in the United States, health care, considered a social good and a right of every citizen in the past decade, is now being marketed and sold for profit in a competitive marketplace as if it is a private commodity. In the process, the medical profession is losing its control to an ideology and structure called corporate management. This social transformation of American medicine is the fruit of a history of accommodating professional and institutional interests, failing to exercise public control over public programs, then adopting piecemeal regulations to control the inflationary consequences and, as a final resort, cutting back programs and turning them back to the private sector. The failure to rationalize medical services under public control meant that sooner or later they would be rationalized under private control. Instead of public regulation, there will be private regulation and instead of public planning, there will be corporate planning. Instead of public financing for prepaid plans that might be managed by the subscribers' chosen representatives, there will be corporate financing for private plans controlled by conglomerates whose interests will be determined by the rate of return on investments. That is the future toward which American medicine now seems to be headed. (Starr 1984:449)

The current policies and structure of the American health care system fosters this dire prediction, which obviously moves further away from a PHC ideology and structure and toward a system that, when translated to the community level, will foster and increase inequality. It seems ironic that the report of the president's National Bipartisan Commission on Central America states that "the United States can play an important role in supporting Central American efforts to achieve adequate and comprehensive health care. The immediate priorities of such a program are the eradication of malnutrition, the provision of primary health care, the prevention of disease, the improvement of health delivery systems, the development of adequate secondary and tertiary backup institutions (improving those that already exist–building anew only when essential) and the training of health manpower" (1983:90–91). In order to accomplish these objectives, they recommend the expansion of technical assistance programs by AID, and that a regional center be established (either in Costa Rica or Panama) to train health care workers.

On the other hand, the Costa Rican system is structured for increased equality and thus leaves one with a more optimistic outlook for the development of PHC, although the linkages of the various levels of the system are tied to the International Monetary System. Thus, in one country, the United States, the problems of implementing PHC are structural and ideological, while in Costa Rica, the problems are structural and economic. As Guerrero (1983) points out, both developed and lesser-developed countries need to find a means to increase coverage of health services and to reduce cost. Both systems still foster a curative rather than a preventive model of health care service delivery, and consequently, medical professionals need to be exposed to the concepts of PHC and not remain indifferent to health care beyond medicine (Salgado 1984). Alford feels "that there is a reasonably high correlation between ideologies and personal incentives of doctors, researchers, administrators and the organizational interests of the medical profession, hospitals, or public health association" (1975:21).

The policies of both countries will have to contend with the dominant ideology of the medical profession as well as the three perspectives that, according to Alford (1972) have affected health policy in the United States—market reformers, equal rights reformers, and bureaucratic reformers. Balancing these forces within the ideology of PHC and a capitalistic system (which presents a conflict between the present health system and the pursuit of profit) will prove to be a major challenge to health policy in both developed and developing nations. The health system in the United States is particularly resistant to change, due mainly to the struggle between interest groups (Alford 1975), whereas in Costa Rica the health system is framed within a different context—that of continued threat of revolutionary change; therefore, the struggle in Costa Rica is between maintaining a democratic society while equalizing social services. Health policy in whatever country involves the resolution of conflicting ideologies and goals within the same group and among different groups in the social system and must find solutions to rural inequalities within these dialectical forces.

NOTES

1. The research for this paper was partially funded by Georgia State University and the U.S. Department of Education. I would like to thank Maria Eugenia de Willie, Marlene Castro, Eugenia Lopez de Casas, and Patricia Salgado for their support of my research in Costa Rica. I am also grateful to Ivia Cofresi and Lisa Cottrell for their assistance in completing the paper.

2. Components of a Primary Health Care system (based on the Alma-Ata International Conferences) include the following:

  1. Education concerning prevailing health problems and methods of preventing and controlling them

2. Promotion of food supply and proper nutrition
3. An adequate supply of safe water and basic sanitation
4. Maternal and child health care, including family planning
5. Immunization against the major infectious diseases
6. Prevention and control of locally endemic diseases
7. Appropriate treatment of common diseases and injuries
8. Provision of essential drugs

Integrating Traditional and Western Medicine in the People's Republic of China: Policy Issues in Socio-Historical Context

Peter Kong-ming New and Yuet Wah Cheung

When the Thirtieth World Health Assembly met, the member countries decided that the major goal to be achieved would be "the attainment by all citizens of the world by the year 2000 of a health that will permit them to lead a socially and economically productive life" (World Health Organization 1983a). The following year, 1978, 134 countries met in Alma-Ata, USSR, to further this goal, by stressing that adequate primary health care was the primary ingredient. In order to encourage all countries to move along these lines, WHO and UNICEF passed resolutions that indigenous health workers (traditional healers, herbalists, midwives, and other folk healers) should be integrated into the total delivery system (World Health Organization and UNICEF 1978).[1] A second conference on primary health care was held in Yexian County, Shandong Province, China, in 1982 (World Health Organization 1983b). China became the unique setting for this second meeting for a variety of reasons. In recent years, China has always been held up as the prime example of a country where traditional and Western medicine has truly been integrated. WHO and UNICEF felt that this was, therefore, an excellent setting to examine, firsthand, how health manpower was utilized, how the people became involved in their own health care, and how this "success story" was financed. After two weeks of close examination of the pieces and parts, the officials of this conference were well impressed by the system and felt that other nations should take a lesson from China and work harder to achieve their goals.

Although the report did go into some detail as to how the various components of health care in China did or did not work, the short report could not cover all the subtle and not-so-subtle underpinnings (i.e., socio-historical forces, cultural practices, and political ramifications, just to name a few) which resulted in the current state of health care. There have been other, more immediate and pressing shifts of policy in China, since the death of Chairman Mao in 1976, which may slowly dismantle the present articulation between traditional and Western medicine. These forces were not considered by the WHO participants in China.

However, this paper is not intended to point out the shortcomings of the report. In another paper, Pillsbury (1982) has already presented a remarkably thorough analysis of the reasons most nations encountered difficulties in implementing the high ideals of WHO which encouraged an "integrated" push toward health care for all by utilizing traditional and Western medicine. Basically, she mentioned that the success or failure of combining the two approaches must consider "the linkage . . . between the narrower issues concerning traditional practitioners . . . and the much broader bureaucratic, professional, and policy issues constraining, or at least concerning, entire programs" (1982:1828).

In this paper, we wish to focus on some of the broader bureaucratic, professional, and policy issues *in their historical contexts,* which ultimately led the current government to integrate traditional and Western medicine in its attempt to deliver comprehensive primary health care to everyone. In our consideration, we will pay attention to the tug-of-war between the traditional healers and the Western-trained physicians who represented the modern, scientific approach. Even after the Communists came into power, the desire of Chairman Mao to integrate traditional and Western medicine did not come easily. More recently, even when the WHO participants were in China for the primary health care conference, there were signs that the integrated system may be in some danger. We begin with a brief history of the introduction of Western medicine into China by the medical missionaries.

MISSIONARY MEDICINE

Traditional medicine in China existed for thousands of years before Western medicine came to its shores (Unschuld 1982).[2] Until the 1800s, Westerners were not allowed to live and work in China. The country was not influenced to any large extent by Western ideas, much less science and technology (Buck 1980). Medical missionaries began to make some inroads, primarily through the southern port city of Guanzhou. Within a few short years after Peter Parker, B.D., M.D., first stepped foot in China in 1834 (Gulick 1973), other medical missionaries also arrived in China. In 1838, this small group established the Medical Missionary Society in China (Wong and Wu 1973:318). One might add that the American Medical Association did not start until 1847. These missionaries came mainly from the United Kingdom and the United States, with a few others from Canada and other European countries. But they never numbered much over six hundred at any time (Cheung 1982:52–60).

As missionaries, in general, grew larger in numbers, the medical missionaries were able to expand their activities—they built hospitals, clinics, medical schools, nursing schools, medical technology schools, etc. (Cheung and New 1983; New and Cheung 1984b). In time, they succeeded in convincing youths in China that the study of medicine was just as important as the study of classics, and gradually some even went abroad to the United Kingdom, the United States, Canada, and elsewhere to study (Buck 1980:8–90). By 1915, sufficient numbers of Western-trained Chinese physicians had begun to practice to start the National Medical Association (Wong and Wu 1973:604). In 1925, the Medical Missionary Society in China (which had already changed its name to the China Medical Missionary Association) became the China Medical Association (Wong and Wu 1973:674). On April 15, 1932, that association and the National Medical Association merged to become the Chinese Medical Association, with Way-sung New, M.D., as its first president. The first meeting, significantly, had 450 delegates, of whom 107 were foreigners (Wong and Wu 1973:774).

Throughout this period of steady growth and influence of Western medicine, the stress was on "modern" medicine and public health. Persons who were eligible to join the National Medical Association, when it first began, had to be graduates of "recognized foreign universities or colleges" or graduates from medical colleges in China which were "recognized" by the association and who had a "good reading and writing knowledge of at least one western language." Others who did not meet these qualifications could be associate members (Wong and Wu 1973:605).

HOW TRADITIONAL MEDICINE WAS ORGANIZED

By 1915, a strong Western influence in medicine had already appeared in China. Traditional Chinese healers were not as well organized. As far back as A.D. 1076, an Imperial Medical College was founded mainly to serve the imperial households, although in A.D. 1166, this college was disbanded; but it was reestablished in A.D. 1191 (Wong and Wu 1973:94). Medicine, surgery, and acupuncture were the major topics of those days. Examinations were given to test the clinical skills of the students as well as their knowledge of theory, including differential diagnosis by the pulse, prescriptions and therapeutics, clinical medicine and surgery, and the influence of the air and the stars (Wong and Wu 1973:95). Those who passed with the highest grades were given official appointments or ordered to compile and write medical books, or engaged as teachers. The "second grade" graduates were given licenses to practice. The "not satisfactory" graduates had to repeat, while those who failed were ordered not to enter that profession and to change to some other work (Wong and Wu 1973:95). During the Yuan dynasty (1279–1368), the *t'ai-i-yuan* or the College of Imperial Physicians was founded. The college had administrative powers to "direct all medical matters, to dispense medicines for the imperial household and to supervise the work of medical officers" (Wong and Wu 1973:133). The state of Chinese medicine reached its nadir in the Ming dynasty (1368–1644) when many Japanese came to China to study. Upon their return, they would write about and practice Chinese medicine in Japan (Wong and Wu 1973:136). Although the Imperial Colleges of Medicine flourished and their influence went beyond China's boundaries, the practitioners themselves never organized for mutual improvement and monitoring of their own activities.

Toward the end of the Ming dynasty and the beginning of the Qing dynasty (1644–1911), traditional Chinese medicine began to decline. Only one Imperial College of Physicians remained, in Beijing, and it was only maintained for the imperial household. No rules and regulations governed the practice of Chinese medicine, and anyone could set up a practice.

Various "schools" of thought and practice also sprang up, led by certain distinguished physicians of that period (Wong and Wu 1973:142). This was certainly analogous to what was happening in the United States, which had many "schools," such as the botanics, eclectics, Thomsonians, homeopaths, chiropractors, and osteopaths, among others in that same period (see Duffy 1976). The "schools" in China advocated the use of "strong" and "weak" medicines (Wong and Wu 1973:143), again reminiscent of the strong purgatives and weak emetics used in the United States in that same time. The strong drugs were used in northern China, while the weak drugs were used in the south, around Jiangsu and Zhejiang provinces.

THE SLIDE INTO NEAR-OBLIVION

By 1869, according to an account given by J. Dudgeon, M.D., the Imperial College had become moribund. China, itself, was beginning to be concerned about its place in the world: "After the Sino-Japanese and the Russo-Japanese Wars, China was rudely awakened to the fact that she was far behind the times especially in the matter of guns, battleships, industries, government, organization, scientific achievements, etc." (Wong and Wu 1973:143).

Several factors, then, came together to force traditional Chinese medicine into further decline. The Qing dynasty was coming to an end. At the same time, Western-trained Chinese physicians and medical missionaries seemed to have formed a powerful alliance to push Western medicine into the fore. Traditional medicine, not well organized, was easily pushed aside. Organized Western medical groups also exerted a fair amount of influence on the newly formed Chinese government.

A hint that the traditional Chinese physicians had indeed lost power came in 1914 when Wang Ta-hiseh, minister of education at that time, refused a request by representatives of traditional practitioners to register their medical society (Wong and Wu 1973:159–68). These practitioners hastily organized the Medical Salvation Committee, which once again petitioned the government, but again to no avail. The Board of Education, in fact, stated that it chose to side with a modern medical curriculum. On September 30, 1915, a presidential mandate was issued to give recognition to "new medicine," meaning a Western scientific curriculum. In February 1922, the Ministry of Interior went further and promulgated a series of regulations to govern the practice of traditional medicine. Various traditional medical organizations sprang up to object to this new ruling, and, for the moment, the ministry agreed to delay the promulgation of these rules.

FURTHER SETBACKS

Three years later, in 1925, the Society for the Advancement of Education met in Shanxi Province to deliberate various new measures in education which should be put in force. The Jiangsu Native Medical Society proposed that traditional medicine should be taught in schools recognized by the Board of Education. This was adopted. In 1925, the educational associations of Zhejiang and Hubei provinces proposed a similar resolution at the National Education Conference held in Hankow, and it also passed. The National Medical Association and its allies circulated a petition among all provincial educational associations that only Western medicine should be recognized, and this effectively delayed the ministry from enacting the earlier resolutions which were passed.

On November 1, 1928, the Ministry of Health was finally established in Nanjing, the capital. At the first conference of the National Board of Health, February 25, 1929, a group of Western-trained Chinese physicians, representing the various associations and universities, petitioned the ministry to abolish traditional medicine. This Resolution for Abolishing the Native Practice advanced four reasons:

1. The old-style medicine of China adopts the doctrines of the Ying Yang Principle, the five elements, the six atmospheres, the viscera and the course of blood vessels. These are pure speculations having not a grain of truth.
2. In diagnosis they (the old-style physicians) depend wholly on the signs of the pulse, dividing arbitrarily one portion of the artery

into three parts—inch, cubit, and bar, to correspond to the internal organs. Such absurd theories are deceptive to oneself and to others. This may be classified in the same category as astrology.

3. Since fundamentally they do not know diagnosis, it is impossible for them to certify causes of death, classify diseases, combat epidemics, not to say eugenics and racial betterment, which are beyond their conception. They are therefore unable to shoulder the great responsibility of such big problems as the people's livelihood and the people's progress and to be of help to the Government.

4. The evolution of civilization is from the supernatural to the human, from the philosophical to the practical. Now while the Government is trying to combat superstition and abolish idols so as to try to bring the people's thoughts to proper scientific channels, the old-style physicians, on the other hand, are daily deceiving the masses with their faith healing. While the Government is educating the public as to the benefits of cleanliness and disinfection and the fact that germs are the root of most diseases, the old-style physicians are broadcasting such theories as when one catches cold in winter, typhoid will appear in spring; when one suffers from the heat in summer, malaria will come in autumn. These reactionary thoughts are the greatest hindrance to scientific progress. (Wong and Wu 1973:162–163)

After these reasons were stated, this petition went on to suggest the specifics as to how the traditional physicians' activities should be curtailed. These entailed licensing and examinations which would include "necessary elementary medical knowledge"—meaning Western scientific medical facts. It also included a "grandfather clause" for those who have practiced twenty years, but they would only be allowed to practice for fifteen more years (Wong and Wu 1973:164). Traditional healers also would not be allowed to advertise, and their medical schools would be abolished. In other words, they would disappear.

THE BATTLE DRAWN

The traditional healers rallied on March 17, 1929, at a mass meeting in Shanghai, with 262 delegates representing 131 organizations, from thirteen provinces. All "native" clinics closed for half a day of sympathetic demonstrations. Editorials and full-page advertisements appeared in many leading newspapers. On March 25, some representatives from this group went to Nanjing to petition the Third Plenary Conference, which was then in session. They succeeded in tabling the resolution of February 25 (Chu 1939; Ch'en 1963).

The Ministry of Education, in March 1929, issued an order to further lower the status of traditional medicine. All "native medical schools" had to change their names to *Ch'uan Hsi So,* or training institutes, and simultaneously, the Ministry of Health followed with an order that all native "hospitals" had to call themselves "clinics." They were no longer permitted to use foreign medicines and instruments. Additional appeals by traditional physicians to revoke these rules were not heard. On December 1, 1929, the Federation of Shanghai, a traditional medical organization, convened a meeting of 457 delegates representing 223 organizations, who attended this meeting for five days (Wong and Wu 1973:165).

On December 17, a delegation was dispatched to Nanjing to see officers in the Central Executive Committee and the presidents of the five yuan. The government agreed to their petition that the status of their profession should be reexamined and that nothing be done to restrict their activities. In January, 1930, steps were taken in the government to establish a Central Bureau of Native Medicine. On March 17, 1930, this Central Bureau came into being. Its main purpose was to "adopt scientific standards of reevaluating native medicine and to improve the methods of treatment and compounding drugs" (Wong and Wu 1973:166).

In essence, this Central Bureau would function as the "superchief" of the traditional practitioners, and its functions would parallel some of those carried out by the Ministry of Health (which had a much more "Western" orientation). However, from the beginning, the Central Bureau's relationship with its branch bureaus and with the existing traditional medical organizations was an adversary one. In addition, within the government, the bureau's relationship with the Ministry of Health was never satisfactorily worked out (Wong and Wu 1973:167).

The Ministry of Health, in the meantime, was reorganized and placed in the Ministry of the Interior as the Wei Shen Shu, or National Health Administration, in 1931. In July 1935, its scope was enlarged and it came under the executive yuan. As far as the regulations governing traditional physicians were concerned, in December 1933, the legislative yuan passed a set of regulations, but they were not enforced by the executive yuan. On January 22, 1936, they were promulgated by a presidential mandate. These regulations allowed traditional practitioners to continue to carry out their practices. They had to pass some examinations, but the procedures were vague, and there were sufficient loopholes for the traditional practitioners not to pay any attention to them. It is doubtful that the regulations were enforced, because the Sino-Japanese War began in 1937.

"TIME-OUT"

While the Sino-Japanese War and World War II were fought, traditional medicine and traditional healers took a backseat to the infusion of even more Western medicine. The Nationalist government received large quantities of medical supplies and equipment through the American Bureau for Medical Aid to China (ABMAC), which was formed in September 1937 (Sze 1944:74). The Communists had also begun their own health care endeavors in the border regions (Minden 1979), and Norman Bethune, a Canadian physician, had a great influence in supplying the Communist Eighth Route Army with some meager medical aid (Shephard and Lévesque 1982). By the end of World War II in 1945, the United Nations Relief and Rehabilitation Administration (UNRRA) provided further help, as did the International Red Cross and the United China Relief (Scott 1977).

THE NEW REGIME: MORE OF THE SAME?

When the Communist government took over the reins of China, it achieved what many did not think was possible. Traditional medicine was integrated with Western medicine. This was the most striking report brought out to the Western world from the People's Republic of China's physicians who came to Canada and the United States in the early 1970s.

However, upon closer examination, this was not really the case—

that is, it took China years to accomplish this integration. As early as 1944, Chairman Mao had asked for a "union" of traditional medicine and Western medicine (Lampton 1977:36), but the Western-trained physicians were still well entrenched and would not give ground. In fact, the Chinese Medical Association, in 1949, still wanted to abolish traditional medicine. The words may be different, but the prevailing sentiment of the CMA in 1949 was no different from the group of physicians who went to Nanjing in 1929. It was, of course, entirely possible that some of the survivors in 1949 were the same persons as those in 1929. In 1949, the CMA outlined five objectives:

1. All the medical and pharmaceutical enterprises will gradually diverge from private and commercial ownership leading to the final goal of State Medicine.
2. The object of medical training is for: Scientific thinking, Spirit of service, and Technical progress—all these are of equal importance.
3. For the practicability of medical training, two grade systems of Medical Center are to be adopted . . . stressing equally upon the teaching and research as well as service. . . .
4. *The unscientific native medicine is to be reoriented and duly abolished.*
5. The patent medicine and drugs for advertisement should be strictly controlled and abolished. (Lampton 1977:27, italics added)

It could be seen that more than thirty years later, Western-trained physicians still held the same position with regard to traditional medicine—abolishment. This was not surprising, since in the P.R.C. government, the traditional physicians still did not have any power base. Gradually, however, through various maneuverings, much too complex to detail in a few pages, Chairman Mao and various physicians in the Ministry of Health and other ministries managed to institute the teaching and practice of traditional medicine as an integral part of health care. Chairman Mao basically took a pragmatic course—traditional medicine was economically more feasible at that time. The famous 1965 directive that health care should be spread to the countryside helped to legitimize traditional medicine. The Cultural Revolution also helped to push traditional medicine into more general use, through the integration of traditional healing into some hospitals and into medical training as well (New and New 1977; Rosenthal and Greiner 1982).

In more recent years, since Chairman Mao's death in 1976, there is a major move toward modernization (Yip 1982, 1983; New and Cheung 1984a, 1984c; Leslie 1974). Policymakers feel that in the health area, there has to be an intensive catching up period, one which would entail a rapid move into specialization and high medical technology (Lampton 1981). As a result of this policy, the government has been making overtures to U.S. philanthropic foundations, such as Rockefeller, Robert Wood Johnson, and others to fund the purchase of the latest equipment and the building of large medical centers in urban areas. This sudden reversal of policy (from the greatly admired health care in rural areas to health care for the more limited urban population) has caused some concerns among philanthropic officials. David Rogers, M.D., president of Robert Wood Johnson, warned the Chinese that such shifts may endanger all the previous "good work": "Many of us envy and admire China's ability to give basic health services to the vast majority of its citizens. You should . . . consider carefully how to protect this system as you transport higher cost technologies when you . . . have limits to the financial resources you can apply to the problems of medical care" (Rogers 1979 in Lampton 1981).

Certainly current evidence points to this shift, as more health professionals come to Canada and the United States to receive specialized training in medicine (New 1982; Yip 1982) and in health technology. The government's official reports insist that primary health care in the countryside is still very important. It still emphasizes training of barefoot doctors (World Health Organization 1983b). However, in direct encounters with health scholars and physicians from the People's Republic of China in recent years, this does not seem to be the "message." If one were to ask them what the status of barefoot doctors is, or how health care delivery is being managed in communes, one quickly senses a reluctance to speak about them. If questioning persists, they would say, "Barefoot doctors are a stopgap measure until we have trained sufficient numbers of qualified physicians." Sometimes, Deng Xiaoping's "sayings" are quoted, that all barefoot doctors must soon learn to walk in sandals, then graduate to cloth shoes, and finally to

leather shoes. They are all being upgraded, and tests are given to all of
them. Those who pass are being elevated to "middle-class doctors,"
and those who fail repeatedly are being shifted to other occupations
just as in the Imperial College days (World Health Organization 1983b;
Sidel and Sidel 1982; New 1982).

SUMMARY

What we see in China since the 1800s is that traditional medicine
and traditional healers constitute the major source of health care. There
were well-organized colleges which trained them to carry out their
work. With medical missionaries and an increasing number of Chinese
youths being schooled in Western medicine and the almost simul-
taneous withering away of Chinese medicine, Western and scientific
medicines dominated China. Medical missionaries, private Western
foundation help, and the Nationalist government seem to have co-
alesced to gain the upper hand (see Yip 1983; New and Cheung, 1982).
Traditional medicine was practically abolished in 1929. The traditional
healers managed to mobilize and block that move. In 1936, they managed to establish the Central Bureau of Traditional Medicine in the
Nationalistic government. The war period, 1937–1945, dissipated the
strengths the traditional medicine groups had marshalled, and the
Western medicine groups gained strength through the various medical
aids that came to China (Sze 1944).

DISCUSSION

In this very brief review of the rise and fall of traditional medicine in
China, one could well ask, Did China really achieve true integration of
traditional medicine and Western medicine? From the information
available of the role that traditional medicine played in the times when
Western medicine had not yet arrived, one could argue that, historically, health care had been designed for the elite. The Imperial College of Medicine was an extension of the imperial household—the best
graduates were retained and only the "second-class" graduates prac-

ticed. If anything, a case could be made that Western medical missionaries were the ones who truly attempted to bring health care to all
(Cheung 1982; Cheung and New forthcoming). They looked upon
health care as secondary to evangelical work, at least in the early days
(Young 1973; New and Cheung 1984b). By delivering health care to
the largest numbers, the gospel could also be heard by all. However,
the medical missionaries became so successful at health care that this
"means" soon became the "end."

In China, private United States philanthropic giants, such as the
Rockefeller Foundation, also contributed much of their money and energy to founding Western medical schools. Missionary and nonmis-
sionary medical schools supplied the bulk of education (Bullock 1980;
Holden 1964; New and Cheung 1982).[3] This became the single most
important effort to foster health care in the Western manner. Their
efforts in China spawned many generations of Western-trained Chinese
physicians, many of whom went abroad for their training (Buck 1980).

These efforts of Western-trained physicians and medical educators
and the large philanthropic foundations combined to overwhelm the
poorly organized traditional healers. Just before the Sino-Japanese
War, the traditional practitioners were threatened with extinction, and
it was only through the repeated urgings of Chairman Mao that traditional medicine was elevated to equal footing with Western medicine.
There is every evidence now, since Chairman Mao's death in 1976,
that Western medicine is again gaining strength.

The case of China illustrates some of Pillsbury's points extremely
well. She mentions that "any national policy may well go ignored
unless a particular individual, interest group, or regulatory body of
sufficiently high administrative authority and capability actively
pushes to have the policy implemented and enforced" (Pillsbury
1982:1828). As we have seen, were it not for Mao's persistence, the
Chinese Medical Association stated openly in 1949 that it wanted traditional practice abolished. Although the number of barefoot doctors
still number some 1.4 million, this is a significant drop from a high that
was estimated to be close to 2 million only a few years ago. There are
now regulations to examine and license these barefoot doctors, a move
calculated to upgrade these practitioners, but at the same time this
move can be seen to lower their usefulness in the countryside (Rosenthal 1982). Now that Mao is gone, there is a general loosening of the

commitment by the leaders to integrate both traditional and Western medicine.

If anything, the shift is now definitely toward elevating the importance of Western health care again. Although the senior author of this paper has not returned to China recently to observe firsthand some of these shifts, when we were both in the University of Toronto we spoke with a large number of physicians from China who were receiving specialized training.[4] From our conversations, several impressions were noted:

First, in order to "catch up" (a current favorite phrase used by Chinese officials) and modernize, China is returning to the former practice abandoned by Mao of competitive examinations. These examinations favor youths from urban areas, upper-middle-class families, and those who had contacts with the West prior to 1949. This means that parents or grandparents who may have had missionary schooling will have the advantage of some knowledge of English, which would enable those who want to go to Canada or the United States to pass the foreign language examinations to enter North American colleges and universities.

Second, China still has limited hard currency. In the health care area, a number of medical centers in China are now placing orders for the latest medical instruments, such as the computer axial thermography (CAT) and other very expensive equipment. To be sure, they are probably quite needed in urban centers, but if this trend continues, the only conclusion one can draw is that primary health care for rural residents will be neglected or will suffer.

Third, in health care, China is again relying heavily on Western experts to go to China to instruct the Chinese in the latest medical techniques. While this is certainly a most efficient way to upgrade the Chinese, one wonders whether the Chinese have forgotten that over-reliance on Westerners, many of whom lack the contextual backgrounds of assistance, may cause greater problems at a later stage of China's development.

In our assessment of the more recent developments in health care, we are not as sanguine as what WHO would lead us to believe. In China, there are signs that benign neglect of traditional medicine and traditional healers may be setting in. A true integration may still be a dream.

NOTES

1. For more details, see a recent group of papers given in the eighty-third annual meeting of the American Anthropological Association, 1984, in the session, "Strategies for Primary Health Care by the Year 2000: A Political Economic Perspective," organized by New and John M. Donahue. These papers will be published in a future issue of *Human Organization*.

2. The authors are engaged in a more extensive study of the contributions of medical missionaries, private foundations, and the Chinese governments (in the Qing dynasty, by the Guomindang and Communist governments) in Western health care. See their reports: Cheung 1982; Cheung and New, in press; New and Cheung 1982, 1983, 1984a, 1984b, 1984c. The authors wish to acknowledge their thanks to the librarians and staff of the following libraries for their help in the research: United Church of Canada Archives, Toronto; Harvard University Archives, Cambridge; Yale University Manuscripts and Archives, New Haven; Rockefeller Archives Center, Tarrytown, New York.

3. Besides Peking Union Medical College (Bullock 1980), the Hsiang-ya Medical College, founded in 1914 by Yale University in Changsha, Hunan Province, was another major effort. New and Cheung are presently completing their study of the role that college (now, Hunan College of Medicine) played in fostering Western medicine, under Edward H. Hume, M.D.

4. New was a professor in the Department of Behavioral Science from 1971–1983, and Cheung was a graduate student in the university from 1978–1982. During those years, they had ample opportunity to meet and know intimately a large group of visiting scholars and students from the People's Republic of China. Many of these scholars were physicians from China who spent one to two years in the University of Toronto to receive advanced training in different health specialties. In 1984, the junior author made three trips to the People's Republic of China, and he confirms many of the impressions received in Toronto.

The Impact of Applied
Social Science on International
Health Policies

Abby L. Bloom

The issue I wish to address in this paper is how applied social science influences the health policies of international development organizations.[1] In order to cover that topic, I will first describe how policies are formulated in international organizations. Then I will discuss how social science, specifically applied social science, fits into policy formulation. Next, I will review some of the successes and some of the failures of applied social science and their impact on international health policies. Finally, I will make recommendations for areas where applied social science might contribute usefully to international health policy formulation during the next few years.

THE POLICY PROCESS IN INTERNATIONAL ORGANIZATIONS

Very few anthropologists have been involved in mainstream international health policy. In fact, I do not know of any beyond the policy office within the Agency for International Development where anthropologists are involved in policy development on an institutionalized basis. The term "policy," however, has been narrowly defined in the literature (Ukeles 1977; Mullhauser 1975) and, therefore, does not perfectly fit the tasks of the anthropologists who work in the international policy arena. The policy process in international health involves five distinct tasks.

Policy research, the first task, can involve in-house research, review of the academic literature, and review of evaluative research on development programs. It can also involve contracting out academic research, applied research that is actually performed by people not in the direct employ of the development organization commissioning the work.

The second task, policy analysis, involves the review of material with the strategic aim of determining what specific issues or areas will be of particular importance in the future (that is, what areas should be addressed in the next three to five years). Another term for this task is "strategic analysis." It involves synthesizing facts and information and coming to conclusions about what might happen in the future and what position a particular organization should take with regard to those potential events.

The next task is policy formulation itself, which involves, as one might expect, the actual determination and writing of policies. That is done in a variety of ways, both formal and informal. Most large international organizations have sectorial policies, such as health policies, and each has a formal document which sets forth its positions. But in addition to that, there are often informal ways in which policy is formulated. For example, the head of a major organization will be giving a major speech, with perhaps a worldwide audience. Policy can be formulated in the process of writing that speech, putting into the speech certain interpretations, expectations, commitments, or emphases which cause an evolution in the formal policy. Similarly, policy can be formulated in the interplay between the United States Congress and the agencies where policies originate but are later articulated or interpreted in response to queries from Congress.

The fourth task in policy is the publication or dissemination of specific policies and strategies. This is done in a variety of ways: through the formal policy documents which are widely distributed; through informal statements in speeches, letters to the editors of major newspapers, etc.; and in responses to queries either from congressional interests or from individual citizens.

Finally, a very important task in policymaking is the enforcement of policy. This is done to a lesser or to a greater degree by different organizations. One of the features that distinguishes policy development in the Agency for International Development is that the enforcement of policy is done by the same part of the agency that actually determines what those policies are. What does that mean in practice? The unit that is responsible for policy formation in AID also has responsibility for determining how the budget is spent, how it is distributed among different countries, and for what specific or sectorial purposes. That means that rather than being an ivory-tower pursuit, policy can be backed by the power of the purse string. It is the power to actually veto proposed projects or ways of spending money that makes policy a potent force in that agency as opposed to many others. In the U.S. Agency for International Development, those who are responsible for policy have traditionally had an additional responsibility, that of reviewing every significant proposed project that comes in from the field—in the case of health, that may be thirty projects a year—for consistency with policy, and, if necessary, determining that the project should not be approved because it is inconsistent with agency policy.

APPLIED SOCIAL SCIENCE AND POLICY FORMULATION

So far, I have referred mainly to the U.S. Agency for International Development because it is the organization with which I am familiar. Also, I believe it to be the organization which has been most cognizant of and most receptive to the important role of applied social science in development policy. What about other development organizations? When I was preparing this paper, I interviewed a number of people with policy responsibilities in other international organizations, and I asked the head of the health, population, and nutrition office of a major organization, "What, if any, impact has applied social science had on health policy?" His answer was swift and unequivocal. "None whatsoever." In most cases the role of the social scientist with regard to health, domestic water, and sanitation programs is that of a very concerned and committed individual on the fringes of the decision-making process, trying frantically to get the attention of decision makers. This role has been described by another author as that of "a shrieking harpy on the sidelines." That may be an exaggeration, but I think it is often true that the social scientists' opinions and advice are the last to be sought (Bernard 1974; Caplan 1979a and 1979b).

It is undoubtedly true, however, that in many instances applied social science has had some impact on international health policies. But this is often as an afterthought. Sometimes the process may be serendipitous— "Oh, let's get a social scientist on the team"—though he or she is usually seen as the most expendable and therefore the first to go if funding is short, and his or her advice is usually given least credence. Alternatively, when it becomes patently obvious that some development project is not working, the reaction may be: "What a mess. We need a social scientist to diagnose the source of the problem." Or, in the case of a health project: "Few people are using our new health services, something must be wrong. Maybe we ought to call in a social scientist and have him find out why. Nothing elaborate, nothing long-term, not much of a commitment, just a few weeks, but let's try to find out why things are not working."

Returning to the second question, how applied social science influences international health policy, it would be useful first to agree on some basic definitions. Although I'm referring here largely to anthropology, social science does also cover sociology, political science, and economics, particularly the new household economics. Applied social science: social science directed toward the solution of some real-life problems. As we've already seen, policy can involve research analysis (including evaluative research), theorizing, policy formulation, and so on. A very succinct but candid definition is that by Geilhufe (1979), who summarizes policy as "advice to government decision-makers on the best way to spend tax money." How does applied social science exert an influence on international health programs then? I'd like to illustrate by reference to the U.S. Agency for International Development.

It is important to reiterate that policy is not a monolith. Policy is made and interpreted at a variety of different levels. Theoretically, policy is the responsibility of a single office within a larger agency, but in fact policies and strategies are made and interpreted in a variety of different arenas. Policy is sometimes distinguished from strategy, which enunciates *how* to go about doing something once you decide, in fact, that is the right course to follow. And of course policy is further refined—or redefined—as it is translated into action, i.e., specific programs. Policies are made or at least fine-tuned at each of these steps along the way.

For example, several years ago the U.S. Agency for International Development emitted a policy that concentrated on certain health sector goals, especially the improvement of financial and administrative systems. One of the regional offices within AID, however, stressed a somewhat different goal which was of paramount importance to them, namely, mortality reduction, particularly among infants, children, and mothers. This bureau issued its own regional strategy which in effect slightly altered the generic agency policy. Similarly, although there has not been a notable emphasis on the use of traditional practitioners in the agencywide policy, one of AID's country offices has been very much impressed by the work of some social scientists and anthropologists on the role of traditional practitioners in a particular African country. In translating global agencywide policies into practice, there has been yet another twist at the program level in this country, where they are attempting to involve traditional practitioners in health programs.

It is also important to stress that much of policy is not formulated strictly from within international organizations, but in response to forces exerted from outside. This is particularly true of policy within U.S. executive branch agencies. In this case, policy is influenced enormously by other executive branch agencies, by Congress, and by the staff of the White House and its associated offices. In short, policy is neither a monolith nor is it formulated exclusively in policy offices or through formal channels.

THE IMPACT OF APPLIED SOCIAL SCIENCE ON INTERNATIONAL HEALTH POLICY

In this section I will discuss the impact of applied social science on international health by examining its impact to date and then suggest some areas where additional social science influence might be desirable. Among the more successful areas in which applied social sciences have influenced international health policies is the area of domestic water supply and sanitation. In the case of the U.S. Agency for International Development, as well as some of the other bilateral donor organizations, emphasis has been placed recently on software versus construction, that is, on human resource development, beneficiaries' or users' needs and their participation, related health education, and operation and maintenance of these systems. Experience has shown this emphasis to be a necessary complement to the construction of new or improved water and sanitation systems. This emphasis contrasts with some of the more banklike development institutions, where the thrust of emphasis is largely if not exclusively on construction, and very often largely on new construction. Social and cultural guidelines are largely ignored, and social scientists in general are denigrated. Why? This is probably in part the result of the professional dominance that pervades any large organization. In this case, the world view of economists seems to dominate in what is a banklike structure, to the detriment of other social science perspectives, such as anthropology.

A second area where applied social science has had tremendous impact on policies in international health is in the emphasis on health care delivery rather than on technology development. This view is not shared universally; that is, many people believe in the potential for discovering a new cost-effective panacea in health that parallels the medical miracle of eradicating smallpox. For example, if we can simply get a better, more sophisticated technical fix, then we can definitely solve the health problems of developing countries. However, the most important health problems that plague developing countries and contribute to high rates of mortality and morbidity are not going to be solved by more sophisticated technologies, but rather by improved delivery coupled with behavioral change. A notable example where service delivery rather than sophisticated technology has been emphasized with great success is in the promotion of oral rehydration therapy. The technology is simple and straightforward. The real challenge lies in changing people's beliefs about the nature of diarrheal disease, changing their behaviors when diarrheal disease strikes their children, and conveying to them the information and the means to do something about it.

A third area where applied social science has been, I believe, much less successful is in community participation. Community participation has been used as a grab-bag term and doesn't really denote anything specific or operational. Social scientists have not done a very good job of explaining to health administrators how to translate the ideology of community participation and the use of traditional health practitioners into pragmatic terms (Pillsbury 1982). Community participation can theoretically mean anything from passive acquiescence to health care services brought in from the outside.

APPLIED SOCIAL SCIENCE AND THE FUTURE OF
INTERNATIONAL HEALTH POLICY

Turning to the future, much greater emphasis will be needed, I believe, in four specific areas. First, development of the client's perspective as opposed to the provider's perspective. To achieve health systems that are designed to reflect an understanding of the beliefs and behavior of clients (and are therefore used), it is essential that this data be added to the demographic and epidemiological data that are usually collected. Further work by social scientists must be done in a second area, the identification of the basic underlying determinants of health status. I refer not to the proximate, medical causes of death, but to the fundamental factors that determine whether or not people live in environments that are healthful. These include such questions as the influence of mothers' educational level on infant mortality, the impact of food distribution in the family on health status, and so on.

The third area where I believe additional work by applied social scientists is desperately needed is in consumer economics and health. We really don't have a very good understanding of the decision-making processes at the household level with regard to health care. In many cases we're not even aware of who is actually making the decision about whether or not to spend scarce cash on health.

The fourth area in need of more applied social science is social marketing. And by social marketing I mean the use of marketing approaches to promote technologies or services which have some socially beneficial end. Social marketing aimed ultimately at behavioral change has proven extremely effective in the promotion of oral rehydration therapy. This approach offers great promise in the promotion and use of a variety of preventive health measures.

The advantages of the anthropologist as an applied social scientist in these and other endeavors are obvious to us but not necessarily to policymakers. The anthropologist is multidisciplinary, though the lack of economic and financial orientation among anthropologists as a group is a severe handicap in the international health field. The anthropologist is prepared by his or her training to accurately represent the client's perspective, and can accurately predict which policies are most appropriate both for client's needs and the needs of international organizations and health administrators. Next, the anthropologist can function effectively as a broker, communicating between the ultimate client and top decision makers and among the myriad levels in between. In international health this involves crosscutting hierarchies among different disciplines as well as different cultures.

What specifically can anthropologists do to play a more effective role? First, I believe that to be more effective as applied social scientists, anthropologists must abandon the professional insularity that has traditionally characterized the field. That means that some anthropologists must work from the inside using the discipline's hallmarks—perceptiveness and cultural relativism—to grapple with bureaucracies as they would analyze any other culture. Obviously, not all can work from the inside, and therefore we must still rely on the talents of anthropologists as researchers and consultants to augment the limited models that currently prevail in most international organizations.

The skills that will be required for anthropologists to exert an influence on international health policies are varied. Obviously, traditional anthropological skills are an asset in understanding bureaucracies, their operations, and how policy decisions are made. Some technical background in the subject matter at hand is necessary. In addition, solid analytical skills—statistical as well as fiscal—are essential for buttressing technical and philosophical arguments with facts that are meaningful to decision makers. But to institute and disseminate policy, a very different set of skills is required. Included are a variety of communications skills, defined broadly: networking skills, the ability to write and speak clearly and persuasively, negotiating skills, and even lobbying skills for those working outside formal agencies (Hill 1984, 1985).

CONCLUSION

Is there a role for applied social science in shaping international health policy? Definitely. Though, to date, acceptance has been far from universal, in fact, some would argue that few in international health today have learned the most basic lessons that Benjamin Paul and his colleagues were trying to convey in the early 1950s, and that need to be reiterated in the 1980s. What has been the record of applied social scientists to date in affecting international health policies?

Mixed. What are the prospects for the future? The prospects are definitely there. The skills of the applied social scientists, specifically anthropologists, are definitely needed in articulating the client's perspective and unveiling the underlying determinants of health, in illuminating the consumer economics of health care and in assisting in social marketing programs. In short, anthropologists need to use their unique skills to thread their way into what may appear to be a hostile, skeptical, and very complex bureaucracy of international development.

NOTE

This paper reflects the opinions of the author and not necessarily those of the organizations with which she is affiliated.

Contemporary Policy Issues in Education for Public Health: Alternative Policy Proposals

Janet A. Strauss and Constance C. Conrad

The intent of this paper is to discuss policy issues in education for public health on the basis of definitions of public health and its practice; information on current location, curricula, and other features of education for public health; and pertinent past, present, and evolving societal values and organizations. Against this background, proposals are made for alternative policies that could strengthen education for public health for the purpose of improving day-to-day public health practice.

For more than half a century, public health leaders in the United States have been defining their field in broadly inclusive terms, while other health professionals, notably physicians, have described the public health domain as relatively narrow. In 1920, Winslow defined public health as

> the science and art of preventing disease, prolonging life, and promoting physical health and efficiency through organized community efforts for the sanitation of the environment, the control of community infections, the education of the individual in principles of personal hygiene, the organization of medical and nursing service for the early diagnosis and preventive treatment of disease, and the development of social machinery which will ensure to every individual in the community a standard of living adequate for the maintenance of health, so organizing these benefits as to enable every citizen to realize his birthright of health and longevity. (Winslow 1920:183)

The 1976 report of the Milbank Memorial Fund Commission on Higher Education for Public Health used a similarly broad definition

(Sheps 1976:3), and Evans (1981:12) stated that "public health policies reflect the cultural, social, economic, and political characteristics of a state." Starr (1982:180), in his analysis of the U.S. health care system, labels Winslow's comprehensive definition (and by inference others of similar breadth) as "down-right subversive," thereby reflecting long-standing concerns articulated by various private sector constituencies about the rightful realm of public health.

Despite perceptions of what public health is, or is not, on the part of many involved within, or peripherally related to, the health care system, it is uncontested that in the 1980s public health practice does encompass an enormous range and variety of activities. Hanlon and Pickett (1984:5) summarize the evolution of public health practice to its current scope: "Public health work has expanded from its original concern with gross environmental insanitation to, in sequence of addition, sanitary engineering, preventive physical medical science, preventive mental medical science, the positive or promotive as well as social and behavioral aspects of personal and community medicine, and more recently, the promotion and assurance of comprehensive health services for all."

Current public health undertakings, reflecting public policy as set out in governmental statutes and regulations, may focus on one or more target populations (individuals, demographic groupings, local, state, regional, national, or international populations) at any of several levels of activity (primary, secondary, tertiary, or "palliative"). One-to-one health services (e.g. maternal and child health care, immunization, screening for disease, genetic counseling, and health center medical care for low-income individuals and families) as well as whole-population programs (e.g., accident prevention, environmental monitoring, planning and administration of statewide disease control programs, population planning, and regulation of third-party-reimbursable hospital stays) are included. The overall goal of 1980s' public health practice is "to enhance health in human populations, through organized community effort, using information and techniques from many disparate fields, in ways that will work, practically and pragmatically, to accomplish what is needed" (Council on Education for Public Health 1980:1).

It cannot be ignored, however, that public health continues to have a less positive, less glamorous, and less aggressive image than that projected by the majority of health professions. Community-oriented responses to distinctive health needs apparently cannot generate as consistently high a level of enthusiasm and support as can private-sector patient care. Quite naturally, this long-standing identity/image/status problem continues to carry over into policies and practices relating to health professional education, including education for public health.

How education for public health, as one type of health-related academic endeavor, is being provided in the United States today, and how it may be better provided in the future, is the central concern of this paper.

EDUCATION FOR PUBLIC HEALTH: PAST AND CURRENT POLICIES AND PROGRAMS

Policy issues in education for public health relate to (1) where educational endeavors are, or should be, based; (2) who is, or should be, educated; and (3) how curricula are and should be designed and used. Policies inevitably relate to other matters also, such as changing demographics and economic and political climates, particularly as these relate to funding for education.

The history of education for public health in the United States has been traced by several scholars who frequently address health policy issues (Sheps 1976; Evans 1981; Williams 1976). Schools of public health as identifiable and accreditable entities on university campuses date from the second decade of this century. The School for Health Officers opened in Boston in 1913 as a joint MIT-Harvard endeavor and is generally acknowledged as the forerunner of freestanding schools of public health in the United States. In its nine years of operation, this school granted eighty-two certificates of public health to fifty-five doctors of medicine and twenty-seven other individuals. In addition, ninety-three special students took courses (Williams 1976:498). The successor Harvard School of Public Health opened its doors in September 1922, three months after classes ceased at the School for Health Officers. Meanwhile, after innumerable deliberations and delays, the Johns Hopkins School of Hygiene and Public Health was formally established in 1916 and opened in October 1918. And by 1922, Yale University, Columbia University, and the University of

Michigan also had established schools. By 1974, the Milbank Memorial Fund Commission was able to identify and survey twenty schools of public health in the United States. At the present time, there are twenty-three, all of which are accredited by the Council on Education for Public Health (see appendix).

The Milbank Commission recognized, however, that by the mid-1970s approximately half of the five thousand degrees being granted in public health in the United States each year were granted by programs in university settings other than schools of public health (Sheps 1976:88). An accurate count of programs outside the schools was delayed until the completion of a 1981–82 study sponsored by the U.S. Public Health Service Division of Associated and Dental Health Professions and conducted by the Bureau of Social Science Research (Holstrom 1982a). Carried out with the collaboration of seven national public health professional organizations, this study identified 317 graduate programs in public health that were located outside schools of public health in 1981–82: 15 in community health nutrition, 37 in environmental and occupational health, 6 in epidemiology, 49 in health services administration and planning, 117 in health education, 17 in health statistics, 14 in community health and preventive medicine, 52 in preventive medicine residency programs, and 10 in public health dentistry residency programs. Information was not available on 6 programs, and a few additional programs were unable to provide all the desired information (Holstrom 1982b:2).

The programs were found to be located in a variety of university settings—colleges of education; colleges of health, physical education, and recreation; schools of engineering; schools of business; schools of medicine; and a few other university units—or operating as consortia of university units. The existence of this number and variety of programs provides testimony to the view that no one of these programs is in itself satisfying the full range of educational needs in public health or offering all possible educational opportunities. The newer programs appear to have emerged in response to felt need and demand, and appear to be surviving by meeting need and demand successfully.

If professional education is viewed as transmission of interrelated knowledge, attitudes, and skills, any or all of the three components may be affected by educational setting. Selected location for education for public health, within the structure of postsecondary education, also can determine characteristics of faculty and students who come to these endeavors and can influence what students will be ready and able to do as practitioners.

Programs in schools of medicine are of particular interest, in view of the issue of public health vis-à-vis medicine. A survey of U.S. medical schools' participation in masters-level programs in community medicine/public health in 1975–76 showed 37 medical schools involved in such programs (Conrad 1978:214; Conrad and Berg 1976). Of these, 17 programs were conducted by medical schools and 20 were based in other university divisions. There were 6 institutions with programs pending and 9 with "other similar" programs. Thus, 52 of the 116 medical schools then operating were involved in some way with masters-level education related to public health or one of its specialty areas, and approximately one-third of these were within a medical school itself.

In April 1983, Berg surveyed medical schools again and reported that there were 28 medical schools with M.S./Ph.D. programs in community health/public health and/or one of its specialty areas (Berg 1983). While this represents a net increase of 11 schools from the 1975–76 findings, it is a gross increase of 16 schools because some of the schools reporting programs in 1975–76 are not found on Berg's tally, and because two programs were classified in different ways in the two surveys (table 1).

Turning to the matter of composition of the student bodies in schools and programs offering education for public health, we find that early in the history of education for public health, in the second and third decades of this century, public health students were predominately those seeking "secondary professionalization," physicians at first, then also nurses, dentists, and other already credentialed health professionals. Education in public health gave these practitioners the concepts, philosophy, and skills necessary to practice their primary professions in a public health way. In the mid-1950s, when federal traineeships were made available for study leading to the degree(s) granted by schools of public health, the student bodies of the schools took on greater diversity, although substantial secondary, or second, professionalization was still occurring.

In the 1980s, however, students who are seeking education for public health appear to fall into three general categories: those recently

Table 1.
Comparison of the 1975–76 Survey of Masters Programs in Medical Schools with the 1983 Survey

| State | 1975–76 Survey | 1983 Survey | | |
	Medical Schools with Programs	Medical Schools with Programs in 1975 Still Intact	Medical Schools with Programs in 1975 Missing in 1983	Medical Schools with New Programs Since 1975
Arizona				Arizona
California	Stanford	Stanford		Southern California
Colorado	Colorado		Colorado	
Connecticut	Yale		Yale (classified as school of public health)	Connecticut
D.C.		Georgetown (was called "other similar" in 1975)		Howard
Georgia	Emory	Emory		
Illinois	Northwestern	Northwestern		
Indiana	Indiana		Indiana	

Iowa	Iowa	Iowa		Iowa
Maryland				Maryland
Minnesota				Minnesota
Mississippi	Mississippi	Mississippi		
Missouri	Missouri	Missouri		
New Jersey				Rutgers
New York	State Univ. of Albany Rochester State Univ. at Buffalo	Rochester State Univ. at Buffalo	Albany Med. College of Union University	N.Y. Med. College at Valhalla New York Univ.
Ohio	Ohio State	Ohio State		Case Western Res.
Pennsylvania	Med. College of Pa.		Med. College of Pa.	
Tennessee	Meharry		Meharry*	
Utah	Utah	Utah		
West Virginia				Marshall Univ.
Wisconsin	Wisconsin-Madison	Wisconsin-Madison		Wisconsin-Milwaukee
Totals	17	12	6	16

*After the presentation of this paper, this classification was discovered to be due to a failure in reporting, not an absence of the Meharry program.

graduated from baccalaureate programs who have no work experience, some of whom continue their education because of the tight employment market; those with or without master's or doctoral degrees who have had work experience outside the field of public health, who wish to change career direction; and those with or without graduate degrees who have had public health experience in entry-level, mid-level, or executive-level positions and who are seeking initial or additional public health academic credentials.

Because the practice of public health follows various paths, with application of varied problem-solving skills and ideas from many disciplines, it is natural that public health students come from varied undergraduate and professional backgrounds. Data for 1978–79 show that among the 3,735 students in the twenty then-existing schools of public health, 10.5 percent had the M.D. degree, 16.4 percent had a nonpublic health masters degree, and 4.2 percent had a nonpublic health doctoral degree other than the M.D. Of this same student group, 54.4 percent had had health-related work experience and 28.8 percent had had other work experience (Bureau of Health Professions 1982:315). Exactly comparable data have not been amassed for the total number of students in public health programs outside the schools of public health, although similar data are represented by type of program in the 1982 report on the Bureau of Social Science Research study. And the summary section of this report states that "very few appeared to have come to their graduate studies directly from undergraduate school. The highest proportion of those reported as students prior to enrollment in graduate programs was in community health nutrition and environmental and occupational health programs (about 25 percent each)" (Holstrom 1982a:167). Obviously, the diversity in student bodies, as well as the range of activities in public health practice, mandate both currency and flexibility in public health curricula.

The variety of professional roles that need to be carried out in effective public health agencies require that an elaborate curricular menu, or set of menus, be offered in the various educational settings already noted. Although all offerings cannot be made available in each and every setting, the student of public health needs to be prepared for anticipation of, prevention of, and responsiveness to public health problems. For the past ten to twelve years, content of public health curricula has been characterized by core course work intended to convey the breadth of public health, supplemented by public health specialty and sub-specialty courses which provide in-depth knowledge and skills necessary to public health practice.

The Milbank Commission identified "a knowledge base for public health" composed of two types of content. The first "includes three elements, central and generic to public health . . .: 1. the measurement and analytic sciences of epidemiology and biostatistics; 2. social policy and the history and philosophy of public health; 3. the principles and practice of management and organization for public health"; the second, "a group of cognate disciplines which are, in various combinations, often fundamental to the understanding of public health problems" (Sheps 1976:60).

In each school of public health, a core curriculum embraces the essentials of this knowledge base, in some cases in one overview course or series of courses, in others in a set of courses each of which deals with a segment of the knowledge base. The Association of Schools of Public Health (ASPH) is currently undertaking a study of core subject areas and has appointed work groups to assess the body of knowledge needed by public health graduates in the several core subject areas and to formulate recommendations concerning the core elements of public health curricula.

Specialty courses generally come within the subject areas of epidemiology and biostatistics (the two basic public health sciences/disciplines), environmental and occupational health, health education and related behavioral science applications, and health administration and planning. Accreditation criteria for schools of public health call for a core curriculum augmented by coursework adequate to prepare students for practice specialization in one or another of these five areas. The majority of schools of public health also offer specialty coursework, for example, in population planning, health policy, public health dentistry, international health, and other areas.

Public health programs outside the schools of public health likewise offer core and specialty coursework. Accreditation criteria that have been developed by several different accrediting agencies, for community health education programs, community health/preventive medicine programs, environmental health programs, and health administration programs call for various combinations of core and concentration courses. Specialty concentration courses address the particular program's specialty designation (e.g., health education, health administration), if there is one, or provide in-depth treatment of certain core material.

In many of the existing schools of public health and public health programs, as in other fields, curricular content is apt to be based on past conditions even though it is intended for present and future application. Knowledge and skills which have been applicable on the past or are usable in the present undoubtedly will need updating for the future. It has become accepted during the last half if this century that everyone in the work force, including professionals, will require "retreading" at least once, and probably two or three times, during their working years.

Naisbitt (1982:32) offers the following corroboration: "Scientific and technical information now increases 13 percent per year, which means it doubles every 5.5 years. But the rate will soon jump to perhaps 40 percent per year because of new, more powerful information systems and an increasing population of scientists. This means that data will double every twenty months. By 1984 the volume of information will be somewhere between four and seven times what it was only a few years earlier." Further, "the rapid change ahead also means that you cannot expect to remain in the same job or profession for life, even if it is an information occupation. The coming changes will force us to seek retraining again and again" (1982:16).

Preparation for future public health activity, and for lifelong learning, therefore needs to be built into education for public health, probably to the extent of preparing professionals for jobs and careers which do not yet exist as such. Motivation for undertaking self-directed lifelong learning needs to be built in. Skills in responding to newly identified and previously unknown problems, in asking the right questions at the right times, need to be developed. John G. Kemeny, former president of Dartmouth College and chairman of the president's commission to investigate events at Three Mile Island, is quoted: "What we'd like our best students to be able to do is to walk in on a problem they know nothing at all about and by working hard in six months become fairly expert in it." Applying this to the Three Mile Island investigation, he recounted that "none of the twelve of us were experts on all of the problems we faced. Most of us were ignorant about even the fundamental nature of nuclear power. It took *the ability to listen to experts, to ask the right questions and to absorb a great deal of information*" (1980:225, emphasis added).

CURRENT CONFLICTS AND TENSIONS IN EDUCATION
FOR PUBLIC HEALTH

The foregoing cursory introduction to the history of public health
and education has noted in passing certain policy conflicts which public health practitioners and educators are facing in the mid-1980s. The
following unresolved areas of concern need further exploration.

The value of public health practice. The value of public health practice tends to be contrasted with that of the medical practice model in
terms of relative prestige and power. Ideally, since the two areas of
activity clearly are complementary in their applications, the "either/
or" tension between the two fields would give way to a "both/and"
acceptance. Although immediate illness needs may generate demands
that are responded to before, or instead of, communitywide needs for
preventive efforts, the latter must be given a degree of priority in order
to reduce need and demand for curative services both now and in the
future. How investment in prevention can reduce the aggregate need
for personal medical services is a subject for additional research.

The undesirable tension between public health and medicine is seen
with great clarity in debate over divisions of resources. William Foege,
former director of the Centers for Disease Control (CDC) has pointed
out that public health activities are held to different standards for funding than are medical services or treatments (1983:249–51). Although
surgical techniques must be demonstrated to be safe, and new drugs,
devices, and technologies must be safe and effective, public health
activities must be safe and effective plus more. Public health activities
must justify their value annually, in budget requests, and must show a
positive cost-benefit ratio, while new surgical techniques or medical
technologies may gain widespread acceptance and use before such data
are developed or made available. There appears to be an inherent un-
fairness about this method of making decisions, of using double
standards.

Professional roles in public health practice. Do physicians, nurses,
dentists, and other health professionals who work in public health settings become "public health professionals"; do they continue to be
medical, nursing, dental, or other kinds of health professionals; do
they do their initial professional "thing" in a public health mode; or do
all of these alternatives pertain? Is public health a "secondary" or a
second (equal) profession? These questions relate very directly to the

issue of the value of public health practice and they may reflect socialization issues larger than those relating to professionalization. Certainly they represent a fertile field for research in the social sciences as well as immediate challenges to education for public health.

Education needs versus service needs within public health agencies. Within public health agencies and programs there is ongoing need for staff education and training to improve and increase skills and knowledge, and to enhance attitudes of those who serve the agencies' clients. This need competes with the needs and demands for the staffs' provision of services. If there are not enough agency resources to meet both staff and client needs, both groups can be affected adversely. But if resources can be found to permit staff training and education, this investment can translate in real terms to better service for more people in the long run.

Locus of education programs. Another area of tension centers in location of education offerings. The overlapping relationships which public health has with medicine and several other established health professions nurtures continuing argument as to the proper locus in academe for education for public health. Schools of public health vary in location within the structure of their parent institutions, and smaller programs are "all over the lot." Many universities that have not yet established public health programs are unaware of what this field comprises and uncertain about what type of program, or school, would be appropriate for a particular campus.

Funding for education for public health. On a broader scale, support of education for public health, in a number of academic settings, is a public policy issue of major importance. Public recognition must be given not only to the value of public health practice, but also to the need for persons to be trained and educated specifically for careers in this field. Individuals who undertake public health careers are not entering a highly paid field. Annual salaries may not be enhanced greatly by obtaining additional formal education, so students usually cannot expect to accomplish a fast pay-back of educational debts. If for no other reason that this, it is essential to have ongoing public support of education for public health.

Since the late 1950s, there has been federal support, which peaked in the 1970s, for schools of public health. Similar support has not been extended, however, to public health programs outside the schools other than to those that train health services administrators. Although some programs such as those in medical schools, described above, have managed to find alternative sources of support, available funding is uneven for opportunities in schools, programs, residencies, and short-term continuing education and refresher courses.

Quality monitoring for education for public health. As for all educational endeavors, the need for quality assurance in education for public health appears at times to be in conflict with the need for flexibility in curricula and the capacity for rapid response to changed needs. Indeed, the growth of education for public health through programs outside the schools of public health may reflect the fact that it is easier to start something new than to change something once it is established.

Monitoring and maintenance of quality in public health schools and programs is of course of concern to the public, to agencies that employ public health practitioners, and to educators. The procedures now in place for quality assessment include periodic réview by accrediting agencies recognized to perform this function, as well as educational institutions' internal evaluation mechanisms. Accreditation of schools of public health began in 1946 and of programs outside the schools in the 1950s and 1960s. Accreditation standards tend to require uniformity across schools and programs at least in the essentials of location in an accredited institution, curricular content, faculty qualifications and numbers, and student characteristics and achievement.

An example of the dilemmas encountered in maintaining quality control versus flexibility may be found in recent increased attention to toxic dump sites and the expanded need for environmental epidemiologists. Can educational policy keep pace with public policy in dealing with this kind of public health problem? To do so, university administrators will need to address the questions of tenure and the balance of tenured professors against nontenured professors, among other real-life academic problems.

Values teaching versus values evaluation. The sense of a need to permeate teaching with values and attitudes is in conflict with the difficulty of evaluating progress in learning these, and of testing for this attainment. In an environment that seems to be increasingly evaluation driven, if the student is not to be tested, in school or on a licensing examination, then transmission of this content will be perceived by both faculty and students as having low priority.

A recent American Association of Medical Colleges (AAMC) study commented: "The criteria for evaluation of students' performance determines much of their behavior. . . . The extreme influence of what students believe are faculties' evaluation priorities cannot be overstated. Ultimately, this perception molds the values and attitudes of a student body" (Association of American Medical Colleges 1983:15). There is not reason to think this response is limited to medical students. Attitude and value development in students presents difficult measurement problems. The AAMC study further stated: "The evaluation of personal qualities, values, and attitudes cannot be reduced to a set of numbers nor achieved by developing a penultimate form. Faculty must draw on their experience to make 'clinical judgements' about students. These judgements range from assessing how students approach learning and problem-solving to the quality of their interactions with patients, ancillary staff, and families" (1983:16). The study acknowledges that this will take more time for observing students. "The Group stresses that licensing agencies depend upon faculties to evaluate those qualities and characteristics that *cannot* be evaluated by an examination" (1983:17). These essential elements can only be evaluated by faculty and must not be neglected.

Current public health needs versus future public health needs. A last conflict discussed here, though not the last in an easily expandable list, relates to the time-tenor of public health curricula. Are the proffered curricula relevant and realistic, practical and pragmatic, correctly perceiving power, politics, and public health priorities? This loaded question is in competition with the imperative to be future-oriented in the development of new paradigms and creative visions of what should be, and to inspire the implementation of ideas of what can be. Can public health practitioners and educators lead us in finding ways to deal with the demographic shifts that are occurring in our population, the dangers of nuclear energy and nuclear weapons, the health-threatening side effects of new technologies and the new life-styles, and the corporatization of our health care system? Can they envision the future as more than just the extrapolation of current trends, so that unexpected and unpredictable developments will be responded to expeditiously? Is there a way to include both current and future dimensions in public health curricula?

PERTINENT SOCIETAL CHARACTERISTICS—
CURRENT AND FUTURE

Before proposing alternative policies relating to education for public health, it is appropriate to review briefly some of the external conditions which have potential for influencing the extent to which policy changes will be possible.

Our rapidly expanding information and knowledge base. We are in an unprecedented time, when old models of knowledge gathering, sifting, and assimilation seem to fail us. The rate of change has increased, the doubling time for addition of new information has shortened, and new technologies or adaptations of familiar ones pour over us. The influence of computers is still in the ascendency, and computer use is expected to become even more pervasive. All of this creates imperatives for constant monitoring and updating of education for public health curricula.

Demographics. The impact of increasing numbers and percentages of older Americans is becoming more and more noticeable. The burden of large numbers of chronically ill older people (Schneider and Brody 1983:854–55) requiring expansion of both short- and long-term facilities and programs is also reflected in the increasing percentage of personal lifetime health care expenditures occurring in the last six to twelve months of life. The long-range effects of lower birth rates on dependency ratios also will alter our social structure, economic environment, trust fund predictions, and retirement possibilities. Added to these probably irreversible phenomena is the increasing cultural diversity in the U.S. population, carrying with it different kinds of health orientations and behaviors that require special approaches on the part of both public- and private-sector institutions.

The economic environment. A trend toward diminishing tax support for public health as well as other human service programs is becoming apparent. Also, it appears that entrepreneurs are identifying many new kinds of profit centers in the health care industry and are fostering their development. This private enterprise approach had led to "skimming" when practiced in the community hospital field, leaving difficult, long-term care to other institutions. Now we also see local governments turning to private corporations to run public hospitals, in the belief that privately controlled management practices will result in economies that public management has failed to attain. We also are seeing those aspects of prevention that can be marketed for a profit being offered by the private sector. For example, fitness centers, smoking cessation clinics, wellness seminars, and nutrition counseling are being offered at a price which will yield a profit as well as a health benefit. The implications of this trend may be that public health will face heavy competition and will lose clientele for some of the activities which can be income generating. But public health still will be expected to provide these services for nonpaying clients and also to provide traditional free services, which are not profit making, all with diminishing monies from taxes.

Supply and distribution of health care professionals. The effects of the projected oversupply of physicians (Harris and Associates 1981; Health Resources Administration 1980) will be to put downward pressure on other practitioners, especially nurse practitioners and physician assistants. It is expected that an increasing number of physicians will be in salaried positions and working for institutions (Tarlov 1983). There may be some modest correction in the geographic maldistribution of physicians, but other factors are involved in this beyond sheer numbers of providers. The oversupply may renew and intensify the pressures on public health which have been evident ever since the early years of the century when the American Medical Association exerted efforts to contain the activities of public health (Williams 1976:501–2).

The political environment. At least for the short term, there will be a continuing effort to return responsibilities for funding and operating public human services programs from the federal level to the states. The trend to decentralize and to place program control in local hands will continue and will mean that progressively larger numbers of persons, particularly in inner cities and depressed rural areas, will be left out, uncovered by public or private insurance plans and unserved by the more fragmented and pluralistic health care system (Strauss 1975:124–25). Similar cutbacks will continue to occur in federal education support programs and in state budgets for higher education, further reflecting more traditional and conservative political views of the role of government and its human services programs.

The role of the media in shaping perceptions. The mass media, particularly TV programming, serves as a major source of information about health, disease, risks, and epidemics. Thirty to 120 seconds on a newscast can shape the perceptions of the public about the dangers of environmental contamination or their personal risks during an epidemic. Public health must learn how to work with rather than against the media, to meet the goals of both (Curran, Effinger, and Pantel 1983:61). Also, as health care providers of all types take marketing seriously, the advertising component of marketing will be very visible through various mass media.

The international environment. Although we are concentrating in this paper on education for public health as it is offered in the United States, mainly developed to prepare those who will become practitioners in this country's national, state, and local public health agencies, it is important to note the worldwide nature of many public health challenges and the significance of public health problems and responses in other countries.

The world system is becoming more fully realized. Not only can diseases which disable or kill individuals or groups be transmitted from one country to another, it has become possible that all life may be destroyed by use of the nuclear weapons we already have. The interdependencies that this reality entails are just beginning to be understood. And public health leaders are beginning to recognize that they, and all of us with them, are faced with a health and safety prevention problem of a dimension never before encountered. Educating students of public health about this, and their role in dealing with it, challenges us all.

Of lesser magnitude, but still of enormous proportions, are the problems of hunger, disease, and population expansion in the developing Third World countries. Public health and medical problems are linked directly to the pervasive poverty in these vast areas of the world. But already felt and potential effects that these regions' combined human misery and near bankruptcy may have on affluent industrial countries is not entirely clear.

Newly emerging disease patterns. "Despite our arsenal of antibiotics and vaccines, we have recently been assaulted by a series of seemingly new diseases that have breached the barriers of medicine and public health. The serious threat of swine flu in 1976, the fatal outbreak of Legionnaires' disease the same year and of toxic shock syndrome in 1980, and the growing terror of AIDS . . . have challenged physicians and captured headlines at a time when we are celebrating the . . . worldwide eradication of smallpox—a scourge for centuries" (Kilbourne 1983:28–32). Public health, as well as medicine, must constantly be prepared to deal with new diseases, syndromes, risks associated with changing life-styles and technologies, and with unexpected results of exposure to environmental contaminants. Whether or not a particular "new disease" is outside of previous human experience, its current manifestations may require development of both therapeutic and preventive measures not used in the past.

Directly relevant to new disease problems is the changing nature of the "agent, host, environment" disease-causation triad. More attention already is, and will continue to be, paid to the host in this triad (Naisbitt 1982:146). The importance of life-style and behaviors, now being emphasized in the media, in entrepreneurial fitness/wellness centers, in formal education, and in public health programs, will continue to be addressed in all of these forums. Increasingly, the environment will capture our attention and our efforts as information is circulated about the dangers of nuclear power plant accidents, water contamination, toxic waste dumps, and other hazards. Questions about environmentally related symptoms and syndromes will lead to more research, and more victims will seek compensation.

ALTERNATIVE POLICY PROPOSALS

Given the array of responsibilities now assigned to, and assumed by, public health, the history and current status of education for public health, and applicable scientific, social, economic, and political trends, how should public and educational institutions' policies be altered to achieve improvement in availability, quality, and appropriateness of education for public health? Several suggested policy changes will be proposed in top-down order, from those for federal initiatives to those for individual schools and programs offering education for public health.

Federal Policy Initiatives

To lay the foundation for effective ongoing and future policy concerning public health practice and education for such practice, it is proposed that a national commission or task force be appointed. The group's membership should represent all of the major health care professions and providers, the general public, and other affected constituencies, as well as public health practitioners and educators. This group should be charged with reviewing the history and current scope of public health practice and education for public health, and current and probably future socioeconomic characteristics (at least those noted above) pertinent to public health practice and education for public health, and with recommending necessary changes in national policy for these interrelated fields. Recommendations should be formulated, with review-and-comment participation by both practitioners and educators, concerning the scope of public health practice vis-à-vis other health professional practice, and the types of educational offerings most appropriate to preparation for public health practice.

Federal funding policy for both public health practice and education for public health should be reviewed in light of the national group's recommendations and changed to conform with those recommendations. For example, if the study group were to recommend federal funding for public health programs outside schools of public health as well as for the schools, current federal policy would be changed accordingly.

Federal-level mechanisms for ongoing participation in policy formulation by public health practitioners and educators should be streamlined. Periodic review of national public health policy should be conducted with wide participation by state and local public health agency personnel as well as by public health educators.

State and Local Government and Public Health Agency Initiatives

Public information programs need to be conducted on an ongoing basis by state and local public health agencies, to inform other health care system personnel, legislators, and the public concerning the scope and nature of public health practice, the importance of disease prevention and health promotion, and the need for support of public health programs. This information should be used in development of state and local policy on funding of public health agencies and programs.

Information exchange among state and local public health agencies should be stepped up, including all information on outcomes of service delivery (i.e., impact on health status of populations served) and on any research conducted by the agencies. The information should also be channeled to public health schools and programs.

Policy reflected in government statutes and regulations relating to public health, and in public health agencies' goals and objectives, should take into account the advantages of public health's functioning in a "both/and" mode with other components of the health care system.

Clear policy should be established by all public health agencies concerning educational opportunities to be made available to their staffs, including provisions for time away from work and for tuition payments. Staff members should be able to pursue degree programs or whatever other offerings may be available for continuing education and retraining, so that public health practice may be kept up-to-date and future-oriented.

Public Health Professional Association Initiatives

Associations of public health professionals, whether local, state, or national, should maintain active public information programs akin to those of public health practice agencies. The American Public Health Association (APHA) conducts vigorous efforts at the national level to influence policy, legislation, and programming, as do most state and local professional groups with their levels of government. This kind of activity is crucial to maintenance of timely, effective policy.

Public health professional associations also need to develop explicit policy for direct communication with higher education associations, institutions, and state systems concerning the nature and scope of public health practice, the need for strengthening existing education for public health, and the importance of including more content on disease prevention/health promotion in all health professional education.

Education for Public Health Initiatives

Educators in the field of public health must take the lead in providing information concerning public health to the postsecondary educational community to guide the development of policy on education for public health in particular university systems and institutions. An informed and positive attitude toward education for public health must be fostered throughout higher education, particularly where there are academic health centers or other health professional education units.

More public health schools and programs need to adopt policies that will foster innovative approaches to programming, such as part-time and off-campus programs for employed persons, dual degree programs with other units in the parent institutions, granting of academic credit for relevant work experience, use of as many practitioner adjunct faculty as is appropriate to the type and size of school program, and faculty sharing with other university units with appropriate arrangements for tenure credit.

Educators, particularly the administrators of schools and programs, need to keep the pressure on all possible sources of funding for their efforts. Diversity in sources of funding is needed, and funding must be spread more equitably across schools and programs. As noted in discussion of the tensions surrounding the matter of funding, tuitions in education for public health must be kept at a reasonable level and for many students must be subsidized.

Schools' and programs' recruitment policies need to be constantly reviewed and revised to reflect current needs for education for public health. They should also reflect an aggressive attitude toward locating and enrolling students with sound academic backgrounds and with positive attitudes toward social justice, which is widely viewed as the fundamental philosophy of public health. Recruitment of minority students and those with knowledge of underserved urban and rural areas also must be stressed.

Policies relating to curriculum development need to reflect, insofar as accreditation criteria and institutional standards can be stretched, at least the following: understanding of the nature of change and of the kinds of change that constantly occur in the field of public health; a future orientation and motivation for lifelong learning; a public health/social justice values orientation; strong emphasis on public policy and the several social sciences relevant to development of public policy; a research orientation that will foster inquiry into all aspects of public health practice; and content on the growing interdependence of all countries and peoples in a nuclear age—all of this built on the firmest possible scientific base. Curricular and other policies should also provide for education of more public health generalists who can bring a big picture, "forest" perspective to policymaking, planning, and administration.

Basic policy of all education for public health must foster better interface with public health practice. Theories taught in the classroom must be modeled on real-world situations, using real-world data bases as well as knowledge and ideas newly generated by researchers and academicians. Practitioner faculty can be asked to critique instruction for relevance and realism, while full-time teachers/researchers can view practical problems in the light of theory.

The social justice nature of public health, only minimally recognized to date, needs to be acknowledged widely and must be reflected in public policy at international, national, and local levels. This view has not been, and likely will not be, adopted uniformly. It should, however, be introduced decisively into education for public health wherever that is being offered. Intensifying the social science content of all education for public health can help promote the social justice philosophy if, as quoted above from Evans (1981), it is taught that "public health policies reflect the cultural, social, economic, and political characteristics of a state." Graduates of public health schools and programs who carry this perception with them into their practice of public health can do much to broaden understanding of and support for the high value of public health approaches within our health care system.

APPENDIX

U.S. Schools of Public Health and Graduate Public Health Programs Accredited by the Council on Education for Public Health

Schools of Public Health

University of Alabama in Birmingham School of Public Health, University Station, Birmingham, Alabama 35294

Boston University School of Public Health, School of Medicine, 80 East Concord Street, Boston, Massachusetts 02118

University of California at Berkeley School of Public Health, 19 Earl Warren Hall, Berkeley, California 94720

University of California at Los Angeles School of Public Health, Center for the Health Sciences, Los Angeles, California 90024

Columbia University School of Public Health, 600 West 168th Street, New York, New York 10032

Harvard University School of Public Health, 677 Huntington Avenue, Boston, Massachusetts 02115

University of Hawaii School of Public Health, 1960 East-West Road, Honolulu, Hawaii 96822

University of Illinois at Chicago School of Public Health, Health Sciences Center, P.O. Box 699S, Chicago, Illinois 60680

The Johns Hopkins University School of Hygiene and Public Health, 615 North Wolfe Street, Baltimore, Maryland 21205

Loma Linda University School of Health, Loma Linda, California 92350

University of Massachusetts Division of Public Health, School of Health Sciences, Amherst, Massachusetts 01003

University of Michigan School of Public Health, 109 South Observatory Street, Ann Arbor, Michigan 48109

University of Minnesota School of Public Health, 1350 Mayo Memorial Building, 420 Delaware Street SE, Minneapolis, Minnesota 55445

University of North Carolina School of Public Health, Rosenau Hall 201-H, Chapel Hill, North Carolina 27514

University of Oklahoma College of Public Health, Health Sciences Center, Post Office Box 26901, Oklahoma City, Oklahoma 71390

University of Pittsburgh Graduate School of Public Health, 111 Parran Hall, Pittsburgh, Pennsylvania 15251

University of Puerto Rico School of Public Health, Medical Sciences Campus, G.P.O. Box 5067, San Juan, Puerto Rico 00936

University of South Carolina School of Public Health, College of Health, Columbia, South Carolina 29208

University of Texas School of Public Health, Health Science Center at Houston, P.O. Box 20186, Houston, Texas 77025

Tulane University School of Public Health and Tropical Medicine, 1430 Tulane Avenue, New Orleans, Louisiana 70112

University of Washington School of Public Health and Community Medicine, F356d Health Sciences Building, Mail Drop SC–30, Seattle, Washington 98195

Yale University Department of Epidemiology and Public Health, School of Medicine, 60 College Street, New Haven, Connecticut 06510

Preaccredited School of Public Health

San Diego State University Graduate School of Public Health, San Diego, California 92182

Graduate Programs in Community Health Education

California State University—Northridge, Department of Health Science, School of Communication and Professional Studies, 18111 Nordhoff Street, Northridge, California 91330

Hunter College Community Health Education Program, School of Health Sciences, 440 East 26th Street, New York, New York 10010

University of Illinois at Urbana-Champaign Community Health Education Program, Department of Health and Safety Education, 1206 South Fourth Street, Champaign, Illinois 61820

University of Missouri Division of Community Health Education, Department of Family and Community Medicine, TD–3W, Room 137, School of Medicine, Columbia, Missouri 65212

New York University Department of Health Education, School of Education, Health, Nursing and Arts Professions, South Building, Fifth Floor, Washington Square, New York, New York 10003

San Jose State University Department of Health Science, School of Applied Sciences and Arts, San Jose, California 95192

University of Tennessee Division of Public Health, School of Health, Physical Education and Recreation, Knoxville, Tennessee 37996–2700

Graduate Programs in Community Health/Preventive Medicine

Emory University Master of Public Health Program, School of Medicine, 1518 Clifton Road, Atlanta, Georgia 30322

University of Rochester Master of Science in Community Health Program, School of Medicine and Dentistry, 601 Elmwood Avenue, Rochester, New York 14642

St. Louis University Department of Community Health, Center for Health Services Education and Research, Medical Center, 3525 Caroline Street, St. Louis, Missouri 63104

University of Utah Master of Science in Community Medicine, Department of Family and Community Medicine, Medical Center, 50 North Medical Drive, Salt Lake City, Utah 84132

Preaccredited Program in Community Health/Preventive Medicine

University of Miami Master of Science in Public Health Program, Department of Epidemiology and Public Health, School of Medicine, P.O. Box 016069, Miami, Florida 33101

References

Abad, Vicente, and Joseph Suarez, 1975. Cross-Cultural Aspects of Alcoholic Puerto Ricans. In *Proceedings of the Fourth Annual Alcoholism Conference of the National Institute of Alcohol Abuse and Alcoholism* (Rockville, Md.: National Institute of Alcohol Abuse and Alcoholism), pp. 282–94.

Ailinger, Rita L., 1977. A Study of Illness Referral in a Spanish-Speaking Community. *Nursing Research* 26:53–56.

Alford, Robert R., 1972. The Political Economy of Health Care: Dynamics Without Change. *Politics and Society* 2:164.

———, 1975. *Health Care Politics: Ideological and Interest Group Barriers to Reform* (Chicago: University of Chicago Press).

Alkire, William H., 1972. *An Introduction to the Peoples and Cultures of Micronesia* (Reading, Mass.: Addison-Wesley).

Angrosino, Michael V., 1981. *Quality Assurance for Community Care of Retarded Adults in Tennessee*. Mental Health Policy Monograph Series, no. 11 (Nashville: Center for the Study of Families and Children, Institute for Public Policy Studies, Vanderbilt University).

Annis, Helen, 1985–86. Is In-Patient Rehabilitation of the Alcoholic Cost Effective? Con Position. *Advances in Alcoholism and Substance Abuse* 5:103–12.

Archibald, W. Peter, 1978. *Social Psychology as Political Economy* (Toronto: McGraw-Hill Ryerson).

Ashford, Nicholas A., C. William Ryan, and Charles C. Caldart, 1983. Law and Science Policy in Federal Regulation of Formaldehyde. *Science* 222:894–900.

Association of American Medical Colleges, 1983. Draft Report of the Working Group on Personal Qualities, Values and Attitudes, April 25. Project on the General Professional Education of the Physician (Washington, D.C.).

Barkin, David, and Timothy King, 1970. Regional Economic Development (Cambridge: Cambridge University Press).

Bennett, Linda, and Genevieve Ames, eds., n.d. *The American Experience with Alcohol* (New York: Plenum Press). In press.

Berg, Robert L., et al., 1976. *Health Care in Yugoslavia and the United States* (Bethesda, Md.: National Institutes of Health).

_____, 1983. U.S. Medical Schools with M.S./Ph.D. Programs. Report to the Board of Directors, Association of Teachers of Preventive Medicine (Washington, D.C.: ATPM).

Bernard, H. Russell, 1974. Scientists and Policy Makers: An Ethnography of Communication. *Human Organization* 33:261–75.

Black, Max, 1967. Probability. In *The Encyclopedia of Philosophy,* vol. 6, Paul Edwards, ed. (New York: Macmillan), pp. 464–79.

Boyte, Harry C., 1980. *The Backyard Revolution: Understanding the New Citizen Movement* (Philadelphia: Temple University Press).

Brackbill, Y., and H. W. Berendes, 1978. Dangers of Diethylstilboestrol. Review of a 1953 Paper. *Lancet* 2:520.

Brown, J. Larry, and Deborah Allen Brown, 1983. Toxic Waste and Citizen Action. *Science for the People* 15:6–12.

Brown, Lawrence D., 1983. *Politics and Health Care Organization: HMOs as Federal Policy* (Washington, D.C.: Brookings Institution).

Brown, Michael H., 1979. Love Canal and the Poisoning of America. *Atlantic* 244 (December):33–47.

Buck, P., 1980. *American Science and Modern China 1876–1936* (Cambridge: Cambridge University Press).

Bullock, M. B., 1980. *An American Transplant: The Rockefeller Foundation and the Peking Union Medical College* (Berkeley: University of California Press).

Bureau of the Census, 1982. *Characteristics of Households Receiving Noncash Benefits: 1982.* Current Population Reports, ser. P–60, no. 141.

Bureau of Health Professions, 1982. *Public Health Personnel in the United States, 1980.* DHHS Publication no. (HRA) 82–6 (Washington, D.C.).

Caplan, Nathan, 1979a. The Two Communities Theory and Knowledge Utilization. *American Behavioral Scientist* 22:459–70.

_____, 1979b. A Minimal Set of Conditions Necessary for the Utilization of Social Science Knowledge in Policy Formulation at the National Level. In *Using Social Research in Public Policy Making,* Carol H. Weish, ed. (Lexington: Lexington Books), pp. 183–97.

Carballo, Manuel, 1978. Costa Rica and Mexico Generating Self-Confidence. *World Health* (May):26–29.

Casas, Antonio, and Herman Vargas, 1980. The Health Care System in Costa Rica: Towards a National Health Service. *Journal of Public Health Policy* 3:258–79.

Caste, Carlos A., 1979. *Alcohol: Use and Abuse. Cultural Barriers in the Utilization of Rehabilitation Programs by Hispanics in the U.S.*, First International Conference on Substance Abuse, vol. 1 (Phoenix: Do It Now Foundation).

Caste, Carlos A., and Jeffrey Blodgett, 1981. An Alcohol Treatment Model for Use with the Puerto Rican Community. In *Drug Dependence and Alcoholism*. Vol. 2, *Social and Behavioral Issues,* J. A. Schecter, ed. (New York: Plenum Press), pp. 95–103.

Centers for Disease Control, 1982. Report no. EPI–8278–2, March 30 (Atlanta).

Chalmers, Alan F., 1982. Epidemiology and the Scientific Model. *International Journal of Health Services* 12:659–66.

Champagne, Anthony, and Edward J. Harpham, eds., 1984. *The Attack on the Welfare State* (Prospect Heights, Ill.: Waveland Press).

Chavez, Adolfo, 1974. *Encuestas nutricionales en Mexico.* Volumen 1, *Estudios de 1958 a 1962* (Mexico D.F.: Instituto Nacional de la Nutrition).

Chavez, Adolfo, 1982. *Perspectivas de la nutricion en Mexico.* Publicacion L–50 (Tlalpan, Mexico: Instituto Nacional de la Nutrition).

Ch'en, T. J., 1963. *San-i-ch'i Kuo-I-Chieh shi-chien hui-i lu* (Memoir of the March 17 Chinese Doctors' Day). N.p. (Available in the Chinese Collections in the Library of Congress, Washington, D.C.).

Cheung, Y. W., 1982. *The Social Organization of Missionary Medicine: A Study of Two Canadian Protestant Missions in China Before 1937* (Ph.D. diss., University of Toronto).

Cheung, Y. W., and P. K. New, 1983. Toward a Typology of Missionary Medicine: A Comparison of Three Medical Missions in China before 1937. *Culture* 3:31–45.

———, n.d. Missionary Doctors versus Chinese Patients: Credibility of Missionary Health Care in Early Twentieth Century China. *Social Science and Medicine.* Forthcoming.

Children's Defense Fund, 1984. *A Children's Defense Budget.* 3d ed. (Washington, D.C.: Children's Defense Fund).

Chu, N. H., 1939. Nien pa-nien ti san-i-ch'i (Remembering March 17 Eight Years Ago). *Hsin Chung-i Kan* 1:1–4.

Clark, Matt, et. al., 1980. Fleeing the Love Canal. *Newsweek* 95 (June 2):56–57.

Commission on Central America, 1983. *The Report of the President's National Bipartisan Commission on Central America* (New York: MacMillan).

Connor, Eileen, and Fitzhugh Mullan, 1982. *Community Oriented Primary Care* (Washington, D.C.: National Academy Press).

Conrad, Constance C., 1978. Survey of Master's Degree Programs in Community Health in U.S. Medical Schools. *Journal of Medical Education* 53:214.

Conrad, Constance C., and Robert Berg, 1976. Preliminary Survey of U.S. Medical Schools Participating in Master's Level Programs in Community Health 1975–1976. *Newsletter of the Association of Teachers of Preventive Medicine* 23:10–12.

Cooper, CeCilia R., n.d.a. Some Belated Hindsights of a Western Trainer (Honolulu: East-West Center. Photocopy).

————, n.d.b. Program Progress Report Notes (Truk: Federated States of Micronesia).

Council on Education for Public Health, 1980. *Criteria for Accreditation of Graduate Schools of Public Health* (Washington, D.C.: Council on Education for Public Health).

Couto, Richard A., 1975. *Poverty, Politics and Health Care: An Appalachian Experience* (New York: Praeger).

Creer, Thomas L., and Walter P. Christian, 1976. *Chronically Ill and Handicapped Children, Their Management and Rehabilitation* (Champaign, Ill.: Research Press Co.).

Crenson, Matthew A., 1971. *The Un-Politics of Air Pollution: A Study of Nondecision-Making in the Cities* (Baltimore: Johns Hopkins University Press).

Croizier, R. C., 1968. *Traditional Medicine in Modern China: Science, Nationalism and the Tension of Cultural Change* (Cambridge: Harvard University Press).

Curran, Anita S., Avis W. Effinger, and Ernestine S. Pantel, 1983. Public Health: Priorities and Policy Setting in the Real World. In *Science and Public Health Policy 3*, Francis S. Stuett, ed. Annals of the New York Academy of Sciences 403:61.

Current Population Reports, 1982. Characteristics of Households Receiving Noncash Benefits: 1982. *Current Population Reports,* Series P. 16, no. 141.

DeBrum, Justin, 1984. Letter to Editor. Marshall Islands Journal 15–10:6–8.

De Kadt, Emanuel, 1983. Community Participation for Health: The Case of Latin America. In *Practising Health for All,* David Morley, Jon E. Rohde, and Glen Williams, eds. (New York: Oxford University Press), pp. 229–47.

DeWalt, Billie R., 1979. *Modernization in a Mexican Ejido* (Cambridge: Cambridge University Press).

————, 1985. Mexico's Second Green Revolution: Food for Feed. *Mexican Studies/Estudios Mexicanos.* In press.

DeWalt, Kathleen M., 1981. Diet as Adaptation: Looking for Nurtitional Strategies. *Federation Proceedings* 40–2602–2610.

———, 1983a. Income and Dietary Adequacy in an Agricultural Community. *Social Science and Medicine* 17:1877–66.

———, 1983b. *Nutritional Strategies and Agricultural Change in a Mexican Community* (Ann Arbor: UMI Research Press).

Dewey, Kathryn, 1983. Nutritional Survey in Tabasco, Mexico: Nutritional Status of Preschool Children. *American Journal of Clinical Nutrition* 37:1010–19.

Douglas, Mary, and Aaron Wildavsky, 1982. *Risk and Culture: An Essay on the Selection of Technical and Environmental Dangers* (Berkeley: University of California Press).

Doyal, Lesley, 1979. *The Political Economy of Health* (Boston: South End Press).

Drash, Philip W., Cynthia L. Stoffel, and Kevin Murdock, 1983. *A Primer of Behavior Modification for the Human Services.* Behavior Programming and Management Services Series, vol. 3 (Tampa: Hillsborough Alternative Residential Program and Florida Mental Health Institute).

Dubos, Rene, 1958. *Mirage of Health: Utopias, Progress, and Biological Change* (Garden City: Doubleday and Co.).

Duffy, J., 1976. *The Healers: The Rise of the Medical Establishment* (New York: McGraw-Hill).

Dye, Thomas R., 1972. *Understanding Public Policy* (Englewood Cliffs, N.J.: Prentice-Hall).

Elling, Ray H., 1978. Medical Systems As Changing Social Systems. *Social Science and Medicine* 12:107–15.

Elmore, Richard F., 1979–80. Backward Mapping: Implementation Research and Policy Designs. *Political Science Quarterly* 94:601–16.

Emener, William G., 1979. Professional Burnout. *Journal of Rehabilitation* 45:55–58.

Evans, John R., 1981. *Measurement and Management in Medicine and Health Services: Training Needs and Opportunities* (New York: Rockefeller Foundation).

Fals Borda, Orlando, 1979. The Problem of Investigating Reality in Order to Transform It. *Dialectical Anthropology* 4:33–55.

Finsterbusch, Kurt, and Annabelle Bender Motz, 1980. *Social Research for Policy Decisions* (Belmont, Calif.: Wadsworth).

Fischer, John L., and Ann M. Fischer, 1957. *The Eastern Carolines* (New Haven, Conn.: Human Relations Area Files).

Fleuret, P., and A. Fleuret, 1980. Nutrition, Consumption and Agricultural Change. *Human Organization* 39:259–60.

Foege, William, 1983. Budgetary Medical Ethics. *Journal of Public Health Policy* 4:249–51.

Friedson, Eliot, 1975. *Doctoring Together* (New York: Elsevier).

Frohock, Fred M., 1979. *Public Policy: Scope and Logic* (Englewood Cliffs, N.J.: Prentice-Hall).

Galbis, R., 1977. Mental Health Service in a Hispano Community. *Urban Health* 6:33–35.

Gaventa, John, 1983. *Power and Powerlessness* (Urbana: University of Illinois Press).

Gaveria, Moses, Gwen Stern, and Stephen Schensul, 1982. Sociocultural Factors and Prenatal Health in a Mexican-American Community. *Journal of the National Medical Association* 74:983–89.

Geilhufe, Nancy L., 1979. Anthropology and Policy Analysis. *Current Anthropology* 20:577–79.

Gellen, John, 1970. Mental Health Training Program for Counselors in Micronesia (School of Public Health, University of Hawaii. Manuscript).

General Accounting Office, 1983. *Siting of Hazardous Waste Landfills and Their Correlation with Racial and Economic Status of Surrounding Counties,* RCED–83–168, June 1 (Gaithersburg, Md.: Government Accounting Office).

Gordon, Andrew J., 1978. Hispanic Drinking After Migration: The Case of Dominicans. *Medical Anthropology* 2:61–84.

———, 1979. *Cultural and Organizational Factors in the Delivery of Alcohol Treatment Services to Hispanics.* Working Papers in Alcohol Studies, no. 7 (Providence, R.I.: Department of Anthropology, Brown University).

———, 1981a. The Cultural Context of Drinking and Indigenous Therapy for Alcoholism in Three Migrant Hispano Cultures: An Ethnographic Report. *Journal of Studies on Alcohol,* supp. 9:217–40.

———, 1981b. When Socialization Fails: The Crisis of a Drug Abuse Program. In *Children and Their Organizations: Investigations in American Culture,* R. Timothy Sieber and Andrew J. Gordon, eds. (Boston: G. K. Hall and Co.), pp. 179–92.

———, n.d. Alcoholic Hispanos in the Northeast: A Study of Cultural Variability and Adaptation. In *The American Experience with Alcohol,* Linda Bennett and Genevieve Ames, eds. (New York: Plenum Press). In press.

Gramsci, Antonio, 1971. *Selections from the Prison Notebooks* (New York: International Publishing Co.).

Guerra, Fernando, 1980. Hispanic Child Health Issues. *Children Today* 9:18–22.

Guerrero, Rodrigo, 1983. Community Oriented Primary Care: An International Perspective. In *Community Oriented Primary Care: New Directions for Health Services Delivery,* Eileen Connor and Fitzhugh Mullan, eds. (Washington, D.C.: National Academy Press), pp. 104–18.

Gulick, E. V., 1973. *Peter Parker and the Opening of China* (Cambridge: Harvard University Press).

Gutiérrez Ramírez, Amelio, and Frank J. Weaver, 1979. A Methodology for Alerting the Spanish Speaking Community about "El Asesino Silencioso" (Albuquerque, N.M.: Institute for Applied Research Services. Manuscript).

Hall, Budd L., 1975. Participatory Research: An Approach for Change. *Convergence* 8:24–32.

Hanlon, David L., and William Eperiam, 1983. The Federated States of Micronesia: Unifying the Remnants. In *Politics in Micronesia,* Ron Crocombe and Ahmed Ali, eds. (Suva: Institute of Pacific Studies, University of the South Pacific), pp. 81–100.

Hanlon, John J., and George E. Pickett, 1984. *Public Health Administration and Practice* (St. Louis: Times Mirror/Mosby College Publishing).

Hannan, Michael T., and John Freeman, 1984. Structural Inertia and Organizational Change. *American Sociological Review* 49:149–64.

Hargrove, Erwin C., 1975. *The Missing Link: The Study of the Implementation of Social Policy* (Washington, D.C.: Urban Institute).

Harris, Louis, and Associates, 1981. Medical Practice in the 1980s: Physicians Look at Their Changing Profession. Survey for the Henry J. Kaiser Family Foundation, Menlo Park, Calif., July–October.

Harwood, Alan, 1981. Mainland Puerto Ricans. In *Ethnicity and Medical Care,* Alan Harwood, ed. (Cambridge: Harvard University Press), pp. 397–481.

Heath, Dwight B., Jack O. Waddell, and Martin Topper, eds., 1981. Cultural Factors in Alcohol Research and Treatment of Drinking Problems. *Journal of Studies on Alcohol,* supp. 9.

Health Resources Administration, 1980. *Report of the Graduate Medical Education National Advisory Committee to the Secretary, DHHS, September 30, 1980.* DHHS Publication no. (HRA) 81–651 (Washington, D.C.: Government Printing Office).

Hewitt de Alcantara, Cynthia, 1976. *Modernizing Mexican Agriculture* (Geneva: United Nations Research Institute for Social Development).

Hezel, Francis X., 1982. *Reflections on Micronesia: The Collected Papers of Father Francis X. Hezel, S.J.* (Moen, Truk: Micronesian Seminar).

———, 1984. A Brief Economic History of Micronesia. In *Past Achievements and Future Possibilities: A Conference on Economic Development in Micronesia* (Moen, Truk: Micronesian Seminar), pp. 11–62.

Hill, Carole E., 1984. The Challenge of Comparative Health Policy Research for Applied Medical Anthropology. *Social Science and Medicine* 18:861–71.

Hill, Carole E., ed., 1985. *Training Manual in Medical Anthropology* (Washington, D.C.: American Anthropological Association/Society for Applied Anthropology).

Hobbs, Nicholas, 1979. Knowledge Transfer and the Policy Process (Nashville: Institute for Public Policy Studies, Vanderbilt University. Manuscript).

Holden, R., 1964. *Yale-in-China: The Mainland, 1901–1951* (New Haven, Conn.: Yale-in-China Association, Inc.).

Holland, Thomas, 1980. The Politics of Community Action. In *New Neighbors: The Retarded Citizen in Quest of a Home,* C. Cherington and G. Dybwad, eds. DHHS Publication no. (OHOS) 80–21004 (Washington, D.C.: Department of Health and Human Services), pp. 173–84.

Holstrom, Engin Inel, 1982a. *Characteristics of U.S. Graduate Education in Public Health Outside Schools of Public Health* (Washington, D.C.: Bureau of Social Science Research).

————, 1982b. *Overview of Graduate Programs in Public Health Outside Schools of Public Health, 1981–1982* (Washington, D.C.: Division of Associated and Dental Health Professions, Bureau of Health Professions).

Hoppe, Sue K., and Peter L. Heller, 1975. Alienation, Families and the Utilization of Health Services by Mexican Americans. *Journal of Social Behavior* 16:304–14.

HSR Reports, 1983. *Federal Funding for Health Services Research* (Washington, D.C.: Association for Health Services Research).

Hulse, J. H., 1982. Food Science and Nutrition: The Gulf Between Rich and Poor. *Science* 216:1291–94.

Institute for Central American Studies, 1984. Costa Rica, *Mesoamerica* 2:7–9. (San Jose, Costa Rica).

Jaramillo Antillon, Juan, 1983. *Los problemas de la salud en Costa Rica* (San Jose: Ministerio de Salud).

Jones, Charles O., 1984. *An Introduction to the Study of Public Policy.* 3d ed. (Monterey, Calif.: Brooks/Cole).

Kauders, F. R., 1980a. Report on the residency training rotation in Micronesia—October 23, 1979, to January 24, 1980. Manuscript. Department of Psychiatry, Veterans Hospital, Loma Linda University, Loma Linda, California.

————, 1980b. Some clinical and ethical considerations in the practice of psychiatry in the Palau islands: a resident's view. Paper presented at the American Psychiatric Association Meetings.

Kazis, Richard, and Richard L. Grossman, 1982. *Fear at Work: Job Blackmail, Labor and the Environment* (New York: Pilgrim Press).

Kelly, James, 1982. Manville's Bold Maneuver, *Time* 120 (September 6):17–18.

Kemeny, John G., 1980. What Is an Educated Person? Three Experts Share Answers. *New York Times* (May 18): 22E.

Kentucky Bureau of Environmental Protection, 1980. *Executive Summary: City of Middlesboro,* July (Frankfort, Ky.).

Kilbourne, Edwin D., 1983. Are New Diseases Really New? *Natural History* 92 (December):28–32.

Labby, David, 1976. *The Demystification of Yap* (Chicago: University of Chicago Press).

Lagakos, S. W., B. J. Wessen, and M. Zelen, 1984. The Woburn Health Study: An Analysis of Reproductive and Childhood Disorders and Their Relation to Environmental Contamination (Cambridge: Department of Biostatistics, School of Public Health, Harvard University. Mimeograph).

Lampton, D. M., 1977. *The Politics of Medicine in China: The Policy Process, 1949–1977* (Boulder, Colo.: Westview Press).

———, 1981. Changing Health Policy Under the Post-Mao Era. *Yale Journal of Biology and Medicine* 54:21–26.

Lee, Isaiah, C., n.d. *Medical Care in a Mexican American Community* (Los Alamentos, Calif.: Hwong Publishing Co.).

Leighton, Alexander H., 1959. *My Name is Legion* (New York: Basic Books).

Leslie, C., 1974. The Modernization of Asian Medical Systems. In *Rethinking Modernization: Anthropological Perspectives,* J. J. Poggie, Jr., and R. N. Lynch, eds. (Westport: Greenwood Press), pp. 69–108.

Lipsky, Michael, 1980. *Street-Level Bureaucracy* (New York: Russell Sage Foundation).

Lopez Blanco, M., 1980. Some Considerations in Counseling DUI Offenders. In *Proceedings of the Second National DUI Conference. Rochester, Minnesota, May 30–June 1, 1978* (Falls Church, Va.: Foundation for Traffic Safety), pp. 141–44.

Lukes, Steven, 1974. *Power: A Radical View* (New York: Macmillan).

Lutz, Catherine, 1985. Ethnopsychology Compared to What?: Explaining Behavior and Consciousness Among the Ifaluk. In *Person, Self and Experience: Exploring Pacific Ethnopsychologies,* G. White and J. Kirkpatrick, eds. (Berkeley: University of California Press).

Malinowski, Bronislaw, 1944. *A Scientific Theory of Culture* (Chapel Hill: University of North Carolina Press).

Malloy, J. M., and S. Borzutsky, 1982. Politics, Social Welfare Policy and the Population of Latin America. *International Journal of Health Services* 12:77–98.

Marmor, Theodore R., 1970. *The Politics of Medicare* (Chicago: Aldine).

May, Judith V., and Aaron B. Wildavsky, eds., 1978. *The Policy Cycle* (Beverly Hills, Calif: Sage Publications).

McDermott, John, 1979. *Psychiatric Training for Trust Territory Medical Officers.* Grant application to the U.S. National Institute of Mental Health.

Meadow, Arnold, and David Stoker, 1965. Symptomatic Behavior of Hospitalized Patients: A Study of Mexican American and Anglo American Patients. *Archives of General Psychiatry* 12:267–77.

Mechanic, David, 1976. *The Growth of Bureaucratic Medicine: An Inquiry into the Dynamics of Patient Behavior and the Organization of Medical Care* (New York: John Wiley and Sons).

Mesoamerica, 1984. Costa Rica. *Mesoamerica* 2:7–9.

Messer, E., 1972. Patterns of "Wild" Plant Consumption in Oaxaca, Mexico. *Ecology of Food and Nutrition* 1:325–32.

Messer, E., 1977. The Ecology of a Vegetarian Diet in a Modernizing Mexican Community. In *Nutrition and Anthropology in Action,* T. Fitzgerald, ed. (Assen, Netherlands: VanGorcum), pp. 117–24.

Mills, C. Wright, 1950. *The Sociological Imagination* (New York: Oxford University Press).

Minden, K., 1979. The Development of Early Chinese Communist Health Policy: Health Care in the Border Region, 1936–1949. *American Journal of Chinese Medicine* 8:299–315.

Morley, David, Jon Rohde, and Glen Williams, 1983. *Practising Health for All* (New York: Oxford University Press).

Mosley W. Henry, 1984. Will Primary Health Care Reduce Infant and Child Mortality? A Critique of Some Current Strategies, with Special Reference to Africa and Asia. Paper presented at the International Conference on Population, Expert Group on Mortality and Health Policy.

Mullhauser, Frederick, 1975. Ethnography and Policymaking: The Case of Education. *Human Organization* 34:311–15.

Nagel, Ernest, 1939. *Principles of the Theory of Probability* (Chicago: University of Chicago Press).

Naisbitt, John, 1982. *Megatrends* (New York: Warner Books).

National Bipartisan Commission on Central America, 1984. The Report on Central America (New York: Macmillan).

National Institute of Alcohol Abuse and Alcoholism, 1983. *National Drug and Alcoholism Treatment Utilization Survey* (Rockville, Md.)

National Institute of Mental Health, 1984. Inventory of Pacific Basin programs made by Delores Paron for the National Institute of Mental Health (Rockville, Md.).

Navarro, Vincente, 1976. *Medicine Under Capitalism* (New York: Prodist).

Nevin, David, 1977. *The American Touch in Micronesia* (New York: Norton).

New, P. K., 1977. Traditional and Modern Health Care: An Appraisal of Complementarity. *International Social Science Journal* 29:483–95.

New, P. K., 1982. Changing Health Policies in the People's Republic of China: Another Perspective. *Medical Anthropology Newsletter* 13:1–2.

New, P. K., and Y. W. Cheung, 1982. Harvard Medical School of China, 1911–1916: An Expanded Footnote in the History of Western Medical Education in China. *Social Science and Medicine* 16:1207–15.

_____, 1983. The People's Republic of China: A Socio-Historical Examination of Its Health Care Delivery. In *Third World Medicine and Social Change: A Reader in Medical Sociology*, J. H. Morgan, ed. (Lanham, Md.: University Press of America), pp. 173–87.

_____, 1984a. The Evolution of Health Care in China: A Backward Look to the Future. *Medical Anthropology* 8:169–79.

_____, 1984b. Early Years of Medical Missionary Work in the Canadian Presbyterian Mission in Northern Honan, China, 1887–1900: Healing the Heathens and the Missionaries. *Asian Profile* 12:409–23.

_____, 1984c. Primary Health Care in the People's Republic of China: A March Backward? Paper presented at the American Anthropological Association meetings, Denver.

New, P. K., and M. L. New, 1977. Barefoot Doctors in China: Healers for All Seasons. In *Culture, Disease and Healing: Studies in Medical Anthropology*, D. Landy, ed. (New York: Macmillan), pp. 503–10.

Newell, Kenneth W., ed., 1975. *Health by the People* (Geneva: World Health Organization).

Office of Technology Assessment, 1983. *The Effectiveness and Costs of Alcoholism Treatment*. Health Technology Case Study no. 22 (Washington, D.C.).

Ozarin, Lucy D., 1982. Mental Health in Public Health: A Federal Perspective. In *Public Mental Health,* M. Wagenfeld, P. Lemkau, and B. Justice, eds. (Beverly Hills, Calif.: Sage Publications), pp. 30–45.

Panitz, Daniel R., Richard McConchie, S. Richard Sauber, and Julio Fonseca, 1983. The Role of Machismo and the Hispanic Family in the Etiology and Treatment of Alcoholism in Hispanic American Males. *American Journal of Family Therapy* 11:31–44.

Perez Hidalgo, Carlos, 1976. *Encuestas nutricionales en Mexico.* volumen 2, *Estudios de 1963 a 1974* (Mexico D.F.: Instituto Nacional de las Nutricion).

Pillsbury, Barbara L. K., 1982. Policy and Evaluation Perspectives on Traditional Health Practitioners in National Health Care Systems. *Social Science and Medicine* 16:1825–34.

Polansky, Ann, 1981. Extensive Analysis for Heavy Metals in the Middlesboro, Kentucky Area: A Report to the Yellow Creek Citizens (Nashville: Center for Health Services, Vanderbilt University. Mimeograph).

Ponape State Health Plan, 1983. *Five Year Comprehensive Health Plan FY 1983–1987* (Ponape: Federated States of Micronesia).

Presthus, Robert, 1974. *Elites in the Policy Process* (London: Cambridge University Press).

Redclift, Michael, 1981. Development Policy Making in Mexico: The Sistema Alimentario Mexicano (SAM). Working Papers in U.S.-Mexican Studies, no. 24 (University of California at San Diego).

Reynolds, Barbara, 1980. The Unhealthiest Town in America? *National Wildlife* 18:33.

Roberts, Robert E., and Evan Sol Lee, 1980. Medical Care Use by Mexican Americans: Evidence from the Human Population Laboratory Studies. *Medical Care* 18:266–81.

Robillard, Albert B., 1984. *Pacific Island Mental Health Counselor Training Program: A Final Program Narrative and Evaluation Report to the U.S. National Institute of Mental Health* (Honolulu: Social Science Research Institute).

Rodríquez, Angela M., and Luis J. Rodríguez, 1977. Planning and Delivering Alcoholism Services to Cubans in America. In *El uso de alcohol: A Resource Book for Spanish Speaking Communities,* R. T. Trotter and J. A. Chazira, eds. (Atlanta: Southern Area Alcohol Education and Training Program, Inc.), pp. 71–80.

Rogers, D. E., 1979. To the Editor. *Chinese Medical Journal* 92:586.

Rosenthal, M. M., 1982. Health Care in the People's Republic of China. *Medical Anthropology Newsletter* 13:3–4.

Rosenthal, M. M., and J. R. Greiner, 1982. The Barefoot Doctors of China: From Political Creation to Professionalization. *Human Organization* 41:330–41.

Rubinstein, Donald H., 1983. Epidemic Suicide Among Micronesian Adolescents. *Social Science and Medicine* 17:657–65.

———, 1984. Personal correspondence from Truk.

Salgado, Patricia, 1984. Situacion y politicas actuales en el campo de la salud. *Antropologia y salud, cuadernos de antropologia* (San Jose: Laboratorios de Etnologia, Universidad de Costa Rica) 3:9–53.

Schneider, Edward L., and Jacob A. Brody, 1983. Aging, Natural Death, and the Compression of Morbidity: Another View. *New England Journal of Medicine* 309:854–55.

Schwalbenberg, Henry M., 1984. Traditional Economic Systems and Their Response to Westernization. In *Past Achievements and Future Possibilities:*

A Conference on Economic Development in Micronesia (Moen, Truk: Micronesian Seminar), pp. 2–10.

Schwartz, Eugene P., ed., 1973. *Services to the Mentally Retarded Youthful Offender: Manual for Instructors* (St. Louis: Extension Division, University of Missouri).

Scott, M., 1977. *McClure: The China Years* (Toronto: Canec Publishers).

Shephard, D. A. W., and A. Lévesque, eds., 1982. *Norman Bethune: His Times and His Legacy* (Ottawa: Canadian Public Health Association).

Sheps, Cecil G., 1976. *Higher Education for Public Health: A Report of the Milbank Memorial Fund Commission* (New York: Prodist).

Sidel, R., and V. W. Sidel, 1982. *The Health of China: Current Conflicts in Medical and Human Services for One Billion People* (Boston: Beacon Press).

Simpson, L. V., and M. L. Simpson, 1978–79. The Spanish-Speaking Social Service Worker: Attitudes Toward the Alcoholic and Alcoholism. *Drug Forum* 1:339–47.

Starr, Paul, 1984. *The Social Transformation of American Medicine* (New York: Basic Books).

Staub, Michael, 1983. We'll Never Quit It! Yellow Creek Concerned Citizens Combat Creekbed Catastrophe. *Southern Exposure* 11:42–52.

Strauss, Janet A., 1975. Future Trends in Health Care Delivery: A Forecast. In *Report of the Commission on Education for Health Administration, Vol. 1* (Ann Arbor, Mich.: Health Administration Press), pp. 124–25.

Stringini, Paolo, 1982. On the Political Economy of Risk: Farmworkers, Pesticides, and Dollars. *International Journal of Health Services* 12:263–92.

Sze, S., 1944. *China's Health Problems* (Washington, D.C.: Chinese Medical Association).

Tarlov, Alvin R., 1983. Shattuck Lecture—The Increasing Supply of Physicians, the Changing Structure of the Health Services System, and the Future Practice of Medicine. *New England Journal of Medicine* 308:1235–44.

Tennessean [Nashville], 1983a. Oak Ridge Environs Polluted by Mercury. May 8, 1-A.

——, 1983b. Oak Ridge: Mercury Cover-up Charged. May 21, 1-A.

——, 1983c. Freeman Charges Mercury Leak Deception. June 5, 1-A.

Thompson, Frank J., 1981. *Health Policy and the Bureaucracy: Politics and Implementation* (Cambridge: MIT Press).

——, n.d. The Technical Politics of Health Care. In *The Economics and Politics of Health Care*, Engelbert Theurl, ed. (Boulder, Colo.: Westview Press). In press.

Trevino, Fernando, 1979. Community Mental Health Center Staffing Patterns and Their Impact on Hispanic Use of Services (Albuquerque, N.M.: Institute for Applied Research Services. Manuscript).

Trust Territory of the Pacific Islands, 1980. *Trust Territory of the Pacific Islands Five Year Comprehensive Health Plan, April 1, 1980* (Saipan: Trust Territory State Health Planning and Development Agency).

Tsuda, Sally, 1984. Personal correspondence.

Ukeles, Jacob B., 1977. Policy Analysis: Myth or Reality? *Public Administration Review* 37:224–28.

Unschuld, S. D., 1982. Medicine in China. Vol. 1, A History of Ideas. Vol. 2, A History of Pharmaceutics. (Manuscript).

U.S. Environmental Protection Agency, 1981. *Bioassey Study Middlesboro POTW, Middlesboro, Kentucky,* February 24 (Atlanta, Ga.).

U.S. Office of Management and Budget, 1984. *Budget of the United States Government, FY 1985* (Washington, D.C.: Government Printing Office).

U.S. Public Health Service, 1983. *Health, United States and Prevention Profile, 1983* (Washington, D.C.: Government Printing Office).

Valdes, Alberto, 1983. Integrating Nutrition into Agricultural Policy. In *Nutrition Intervention Strategies in National Development,* Barbara Underwood, ed. (New York: Academic Press), pp. 41–46.

Van Maanen, John, ed., 1983. *Qualitative Methodology* (Beverly Hills, Calif.: Sage Publications).

Wagenfeld, Morton O., and Judith H. Jacobs, 1982. The Community Mental Health Movement: Its Origins and Growth. In *Public Mental Health,* M. Wagenfeld, P. Lemkau, and B. Justice, eds. (Beverly Hills, Calif.: Sage Publications), pp. 46–89.

Wallace, Anthony F. C., 1971. *Administrative Forms of Social Organization.* McCaleb Module in Anthropology, no. 9 (Reading, Mass: Addison-Wesley).

Wallerstein, Immanuel, 1979. *The Capitalist World-Economy* (Cambridge: Cambridge University Press).

Weick, Karl E., 1976. Educational Organizations as Loosely Coupled Systems. *Administrative Science Quarterly* 21:1–19.

Welch, Bruce L., 1980. Nuclear Power Risks: Challenge to the Credibility of Science. *International Journal of Health Sciences* 10:5–36.

World Health Organization/Food and Agricultural Organization, 1973. Protein and Energy Requirements. Technical Report no. 522 (Rome: FAO).

Wildavsky, Aaron, 1982. Introduction: Toward a New Budgetary Order. In *The Federal Budget: Economics and Politics,* Aaron Wildavsky and Michael J. Boskin, eds. (San Francisco: Institute for Contemporary Studies), pp. 3–20.

Williams, Greer, 1976. Schools of Public Health—Their Doing and Undoing. *Health and Society* 54:489–527.

Williams, Ralph, 1951. *The United States Public Health Services, 1798–1950* (Washington, D.C.: Commissioned Officers Association, U.S. Public Health Service).

Williams, Walter, et al., 1982. *Studying Implementation* (Chatham, N.J.: Chatham House).

Wilson, Lawrence G., 1981. Utilizing Dispersed Mental Health Para-Professionals for Scattered Pacific Islands: A Micronesian Experience. *Community Mental Health* 17:161–70.

Winslow, C. E. A., 1920. The Untilled Field of Public Health. *Modern Medicine* 2:183.

Wong, K. C., and L. T. Wu, 1973. *History of Chinese Medicine* (New York: AMS Press).

World Bank, 1975. *The Assault on World Poverty* (Baltimore: Johns Hopkins University Press).

World Health Organization, 1983a. *Handbook of Resolutions and Decisions of the World Health Assembly and the Executive Board.* 5th ed., Vol. 2 (Resolution WHA 30.43) (Geneva: World Health Organization).

_____, 1983b. *Primary Health Care, the Chinese Experience: Report of an Inter-Regional Seminar, June 13–16, 1982* (Geneva: World Health Organization).

World Health Organization and UNICEF, 1978. *Alma-Ata 1978: Report of the International Conference on Primary Health Care, Alma-Ata, USSR* (Geneva: World Health Organization).

Yip, K. C., 1982. Health and Society in China: Public Health Education for the Community, 1912–1937. *Social Science and Medicine* 16:1197–1205.

_____, 1983. Medicine and Nationalism in the People's Republic of China, 1949–1980. *Canadian Review of Studies in Nationalism* 10:175–87.

Young, Bruce, 1983. Science *by* the People. *Science for the People* 15:19–25.

Young, T. K., 1973. A Conflict of Profession: The Medical Missionary in China, 1835–1890. *Bulletin of the History of Medicine* 47:250–72.

The Contributors

MICHAEL V. ANGROSINO is professor of anthropology, University of South Florida. His current research interests are in the field of mental health, policy, and community of mentally retarded adults.

ABBY L. BLOOM was senior health policy advisor for the United States Agency for International Development until the end of 1984. Previously, she was population officer for U.S. AID to Panama. Currently she is an independent consultant in international health and is living in Australia.

YUET WAH CHEUNG taught sociology at Hong Kong Lingnan College from 1982 to 1984. He joined the Department of Sociology, the Chinese University of Hong Kong, in September 1984. His research interests include juvenile delinquency in Hong Kong and the development of Western medicine in China.

KATHLEEN DEWALT is associate professor of behavioral science and anthropology at the University of Kentucky. She has conducted extensive research in Mexico and Central America on nutrition and health policy. Recently, she has focused on the nutritional implications of increasing sorghum production in Honduras and Mexico.

CAROLE E. HILL is professor of anthropology, Georgia State University. She has conducted research in the American South for fifteen years and in the past three years has carved out research in Costa Rica. Her current research interests are rural health, migration, economic problems, and policy of women in the communities along the Atlantic coast of Costa Rica.

PETER KONG-MING NEW was chairman and professor of the Department of Sociology at the University of South Florida until his untimely death on December 30, 1985. His primary research interest was a socio-historical examination of medical missionaries in China, 1830s–1937. He was coeditor of International Affairs, *Human Organization*.

Albert B. Robillard is associate professor of sociology and a member of the Social Science Research Institute at the University of Hawaii. His current research interests are health development in Micronesia and church-sponsored community health development programs in the Philippines. In 1985 he was a Fulbright Research Scholar at the Institute of Philippine Culture, Ateneo de Manila University, Manila.

Constance C. Conrad is professor and director of medical student education in the Department of Community Health at Emory University School of Medicine in Atlanta, Georgia. Prior to this, she served as director of the master of community health degree program, now renamed the master of public health.

Richard A. Couto is director of the Center for Health Services, Vanderbilt University, and is currently conducting research in Wales, South Africa, Australia, and the United States comparing coal mining and environmental health policy.

Andrew J. Gordon is a lecturer at the School of Public Health, Columbia University, and a research associate in the Department of Anthropology, Brown University. He currently directs education programs and clinical research at the Smithers Alcoholism Treatment and Training Center.

Janet A. Strauss is special assistant for policy and planning to the commissioner, Department of Public Health, Commonwealth of Massachusetts. She served for six years as the executive director of the Council on Education for Public Health, which is the accrediting body for schools of public health, graduate programs in community health/preventive medicine outside schools of public health, and for programs in health education. Prior to that, she staffed the two-year national Commission on Education for Health Administration.

Frank J. Thompson is professor of political science and department head at the University of Georgia. He served as a public administration fellow with the U.S. Public Health Service. One of his books, *Health Policy and the Bureaucracy: Politics and Implementation,* was recently reissued in paperback by MIT Press.

Linda M. Whiteford is associate professor of anthropology, University of South Florida. She is medical track leader for the graduate program in applied medical anthropology. Her current research interests are human reproduction and health policy.